Practical Assessment

of the

Chiropractic Patient

A Thorough Orthopedic and Neurological
Examination in Less Than 10 Minutes

by
K. Jeffrey Miller, D.C., D.A.B.C.O

kjm@examdoc.com • www.examdoc.com
130 Oakview Drive • Shelbyville, Kentucky 40065 • 502-633-2730

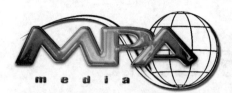

Printed in the United States of America.

First Edition 2002

Miller, K. Jeffrey. *Practical Assessment of the Chiropractic Patient: A Thorough Orthopedic and Neurological Examination in Less than 10 Minutes.*

ISBN 0-9707345-1-4

About the Author

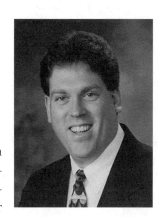

K. Jeffrey Miller graduated from Palmer College of Chiropractic in Davenport, Iowa, in 1987. He completed orthopedic training in 1992 through Parker College of Chiropractic in Dallas, Texas, and is both a Diplomate of the American Board of Chiropractic Orthopedists (DABCO) and a Fellow of the Academy of Chiropractic Orthopedists (FACO). In addition, he is a Certified Strength and Conditioning Specialist (CSCS) as sanctioned by the National Strength and Conditioning Association.

Besides full-time private practice, Dr. Miller has served on the postgraduate faculties of three chiropractic colleges as an instructor in occupational health, orthopedics and insurance claims review. He is a member of the ACA and has served on two state peer-review committees dealing with workers' compensation and personal-injury cases, and is experienced in the review and defense of chiropractic malpractice cases. Twenty-three different periodicals have published more than 80 of his writings, and he is the author of *On-The-Job C.A.R.E.* – now in its third edition.

Dr. Miller resides in Shelbyville, Ky., with his wife, Kimberly, and children Ben, Andy, Emily and Katie.

TABLE OF CONTENTS

Introduction 1

First Things First 3

Required Equipment 6

The Patient Attire 9

Recording the Exam 10

Exam Order 11

Examination Summary and Flow Chart 12

Test Selection 14

The Exam **16**

    Group One Tests 16

    Group Two Tests 23

    Group Three Tests 25

    Group Four Tests 29

    Group Five Tests 33

    Group Six Tests 34

    Group Seven Tests 35

    Group Eight (& Twelve) Tests 39

    Group Nine Tests 42

    Group Ten Tests 43

    Group Eleven Tests 45

    Group Twelve (& Eight) Tests 39

    Group Thirteen Tests 48

    Group Fourteen Tests 51

    Group Fifteen Tests 52

    Group Sixteen Tests 53

    Group Seventeen Tests 55

    Nine Minutes, 55 Seconds 56

Additional Tests 57

Progress Evaluations 57

References 59

Appendices **61**

    Appendix A: Practical Examination Strategies 61

    Appendix B: History and Exam Forms 63

    Appendix C: Functions, Pathologies and
    Corresponding Tests and Signs 89

DEDICATION

To my wife, Kim, and children, Andy, Ben, Emily and Katie.

The differences in sacrifices between a job and a career are immense.

This is especially true of chiropractic, as a chiropractic career

quickly becomes a way of life.

Thank you for your support and understanding of my career.

ACKNOWLEDGEMENTS

Thanks to:

Tom Peterson, Pride! Inc.
for his keen insight and direction in this project.

Sue Schaefer, GetSET
for her typesetting and computer magic.

Charlie Westerfield, Charlie Westerfield Studio
for his photographic expertise.

Don Petersen, *Dynamic Chiropractic*
for his insight and generosity.

Special thanks to the doctors who proofread and offered suggestions during the early stages of this work.

Dr. Barbara Cook
Dr. Richard Haas
Dr. Howard Jacot
Dr. Mark Kestner
Dr. Mark Myers

Very special thanks to Lisa Griffith, my office manager and friend.
Lisa typed this manuscript not less than 100 times and modeled for the photos.
A great job as always!

Finally, my deepest gratitude to the doctors who have inspired my life and career.

We see far because we stand on the shoulders of giants.
– Sir Isaac Newton

Dr. Donald Cooper (1928-1988),
who taught me it was alright to pursue my dreams.

Dr. Russell Erhardt (1926-1996)
Attending Dr. Erhardt's seminars sparked my teaching spirit.
His contribution to the chiropractic profession may never be duplicated.

Dr. William Harris,
for believing in me.

Dr. John Lockenour
John is inspiration by example.

Dr. Charlie Woodward (1929-2000)
Charlie showed me no one is ever too old to learn or improve.

Dr. David Kats,
who provided my first opportunity to teach.

PREFACE

In chiropractic college we were taught to perform hundreds of physical-exam, orthopedic and neurological procedures. After we developed a basic understanding of these procedures, we sharpened our skills in student and outpatient clinics, typically performing every exam procedure we knew regardless of the patient's chief complaint. This was good practice, but for patients it meant enduring a long, tedious process just to get an adjustment. Those patients deserved medals. We owe them our deepest gratitude.

In practice it became obvious that the initial exam procedures had to be condensed. A two-hour exam is not practical in the real world. This left us to ponder two questions: "What do we leave out?" and, "How do we still ensure a thorough exam?" Chiropractic training <u>did not</u> provide us the answers. As in other professions, each of us was left to find our own way. In his book, *What They Don't Teach You at Harvard Business School*, Mark H. McCormack states, "The best lesson anyone can learn from business school is an awareness of what they can't teach you - all the ins and outs of everyday business life. Those ins and outs are largely a self-learning process." This realization is the reason for this book.

Practical Assessment of the Chiropractic Patient is based on my orthopedic training, 14 years of clinical experience, work with hundreds of peer review cases, experience as an expert witness in malpractice cases and a great deal of trial and error. The book is not the final word regarding the examination of chiropractic patients. It will not apply to every single patient or diagnose every case, but the examination process described here does offer a practical, efficient approach that will benefit both patient and doctor. Using seven low-tech diagnostic instruments, the exam encompasses 90 procedures that can help identify a variety of pathologies and can be performed in a 10-minute time frame. The key to using the system is the form I created as a guide to the groupings and sequence of the exam. It will maximize your use of time, and hasten the path to determining the best options for care. The form appears in Appendix B.

Private practice affords each of us the opportunity to develop our own examination style. Do we do a good job? In most cases, I think we do. However, there are still too many cases in which the answer is "No." This book is my effort to assist clinicians in the continued development of their examination skills.

If you incorporate the following examination and principles into your current routine, I guarantee it will stimulate and refine your current exam process. My efforts will be well-rewarded if the ideas imparted assist in providing better care for a single patient.

Fraternally,
K. Jeffrey Miller, D.C., D.A.B.C.O.

INTRODUCTION

The descriptions provided in *Practical Assessment of the Chiropractic Patient* assume that the reader has a working knowledge of physical, orthopedic and neurological examination procedures. The text will not describe each test in minute detail. The reader needing more specific detail should refer to the references listed at the end of the text.

The principles used to develop the Practical Exam Process are identified throughout the text as **Practical Examination Strategies.** The principles will assist the reader in understanding test selection and order. **Practical Examination Strategies** are summarized in Appendix A.

FIRST THINGS FIRST

Always record the patient's history first! Taking a history is becoming a lost art. The process is often abbreviated or delegated to persons with modest training, in order to proceed with high-tech diagnostic tools. This is regrettable, since a good history can often provide an accurate diagnosis before the physical examination actually begins.[1,2]

It is important to remember that history findings determine which physical examination procedures to perform. History and physical examination findings in turn determine which imaging and lab tests to perform. History, physical examination, imaging tests and lab findings together determine the diagnosis. Finally, the diagnosis determines the treatment. The patient's response to treatment determines the continuation or change in treatment and the ultimate prognosis. Do not let fascination with a particular procedure or high-tech gadget disrupt the logic of this order.

There are several components of a complete case history. The primary component is the problem-focused history or chief complaint. This component is required for all levels of history according to CPT coding procedures (See Table 1). Other components, such as reviews of systems, past history, family history, social history and occupational history, are usually added to the case history as the complexity of the patient's condition and coding requirements escalate (Tables 1 & 2).

For practical purposes it is recommended that a complete case history be obtained for all patients regardless of the severity of their problem. This is easily accomplished by having patients complete questionnaires regarding their review of systems, past history, family history, social history and occupational history in the reception room prior to seeing the doctor (See Appendix B). The doctor can then **review this information prior** to entering the room to record the patient's problem-focused history. This requires minimal additional time from the doctor and provides a more complete record. The history is then available regardless of the level of the examination process required to diagnose the patient's condition. In other words, it is better to have it and not need it than to need it and not have it.

Once a complete case history is obtained, the average patient with head, spinal, pelvic or extremity complaints will benefit from the exam described here. The portion of the patient population who the exam does not apply to will present with symptoms and histories reflecting conditions that are often obvious to diagnose (shingles, trigger fingers, sprained ankles) or conditions that do not appear to involve the neuromusculoskeletal system. In these situations, exam procedures must be adapted to reflect the patient's needs as determined by the history. Practical assessment procedures can still be used, if the doctor chooses, for differential diagnosis or to establish baseline findings.

Practical Examination Strategies:

1. Patient history should precede examination.

2. The examination performed should be based on or related to the history obtained prior to the exam.

TABLE 1

EVALUATION AND MANAGEMENT (E/M) SERVICE

NEW PATIENT
Requires 3 of 3 * Key Components

Code	*History	*Exam	*Decision Making	Presenting Problem	Time
99201	Chief Complaint Brief HPI (1-3 Elements)	1-5 Bullets in 1 or more Regions/System	Straight Forward	Minor/Self-Limited	10 Minutes
99202	Chief Complaint Brief HPI (1-3 Elements) ROS (1 or more)	6 Bullets in 1 or more Regions/Systems	Straight Forward	Low Severity	20 Minutes
99203	Chief Complaint Extended HPI (4-8 Elements) ROS (2-9) PFSH (1 or more)	12 Bullets in 2 or more Regions/Systems	Low Complexity	Moderate Severity	30 Minutes
99204	Chief Complaint Extended HPI (4-8 Elements) ROS (10 or more) PFSH (2 or 3)	All Bullets Shaded Boxes 1 Bullet Unshaded Boxes	Moderate Complexity	Mod-High Severity	45 Minutes
99205	Chief Complaint Extended HPI (4-8 Elements) ROS (10 or more) PFSH (2 or 3)	All Bullets Shaded Boxes 1 Bullet Unshaded Boxes	High Complexity	Mod-High Severity	60 Minutes

Adapted from E/M Coding Made Easy, 3rd Edition, by: PMIC

ESTABLISHED PATIENT
Requires 2 or 3 * Key Components

Code	*History	*Exam	*Decision Making	Presenting Problem	Time
99211				Problem Not Requiring a Physician	5 Minutes
99212	Chief Complaint Brief HPI (1-3 Elements)	1-5 Bullets in 1 or more Regions/Systems	Straight Forward	Minor/Self-Limited	10 Minutes
99213	Chief Complaint Brief HPI (1-3 Elements) ROS (1 or more)	6 Bullets in 1 or more Regions/Systems	Low Complexity	Low-Mod Severity	15 Minutes
99214	Chief Complaint Extended HPI (4-9 Elements) ROS (2-9 Systems) PFSH (2 or more)	12 Bullets in 2 or more Regions/Systems	Moderate Complexity	Mod-High Severity	25 Minutes
99215	Chief Complaint Extended HPI (4-8 Elements) ROS (10 or more) PFSH (2 or 3)	All Bullets Shaded Boxes 1 Bullet Unshaded Boxes	High Complexity	Mod-High Severity	40 Minutes

Adapted from E/M Coding Made Easy, 3rd Edition, by: PMIC

TABLE 2

History Requirements for New Patient Exams

New Patient Focused   CPT code: 99201

1. Brief problem-focused history
   A. Elements
      1. Location
      2. Quality
      3. Severity

New Patient Expanded   CPT code: 99202

1. Brief problem-focused history
   A. Elements
      1. Location
      2. Quality
      3. Severity
   B. Review of One System
      1. Most likely constitutional, musculoskeletal or neurological

New Patient Detailed   CPT code: 99203

1. Extended problem-focused history
   A. Elements

1. Location	5. Timing
2. Quality	6. Context
3. Severity	7. Modifying factors
4. Duration	8. Associated s/s

2. Review of Systems
   A. Two or more of the following systems

1. Constitutional symptoms	8. Gastrointestinal
2. Musculoskeletal	9. Genitourinary
3. Neurological	10. Integumentary (skin)
4. Eyes	11. Psychiatric
5. Ears, nose, mouth, throat	12. Endocrine
6. Cardiovascular	13. Hematologic/lymphatic
7. Respiratory	14. Allergic/immunologic

3. Additional Histories
   A. Problem-pertinent information from one of the following
      1. Past history
      2. Family history
      3. Social history

New Patient Comprehensive   CPT code: 99204

1. Problem-focused history
   A. All items listed for 99203
2. Review of systems
   A. At least 10 of the systems listed under 99203
3. Additional histories
   A. All three of the following
      1. Past history
      2. Family history
      3. Social history

New Patient Comprehensive   CPT code: 99205

1. All items listed for 99204 in greater detail

REQUIRED EQUIPMENT

The examination is performed using seven basic diagnostic tools: weight and height scales, a sphygmomanometer, a stethoscope, a thermometer, a reflex hammer (plexor) and an examination table (Table 3; Fig. 1: A-D). An inclinometer for range-of-motion studies also may be useful, but it is optional (Fig. 2). Other optional equipment includes two common forms of examination stools. The first stool is for the examiner during testing. The second stool has a handrail that can assist with patient stabilization (Fig. 3).

TABLE 3

REQUIRED EQUIPMENT	
WEIGHT SCALE	THERMOMETER
HEIGHT SCALE	REFLEX HAMMER (Plexor)
SPHYGMOMANOMETER	EXAMINATION TABLE
STETHOSCOPE	

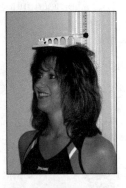

Fig. 1A. Height Scale

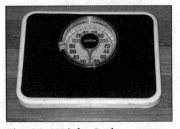

Fig. 1B. Weight Scale

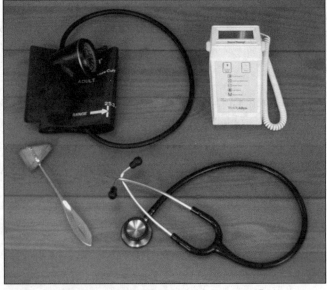

Fig. 1C. Sphygmomanometer, Thermometer, Reflex Hammer (Plexor) and Stethoscope

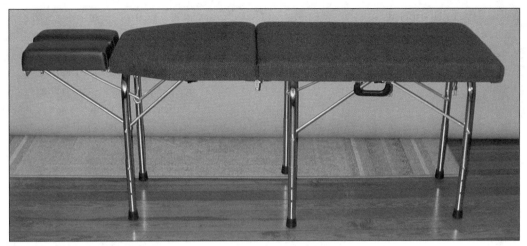

Fig. 1D. Examination Table

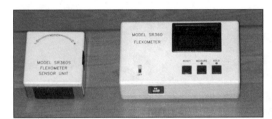

Fig. 2. Digital Inclinometer

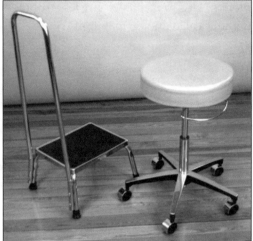

Fig. 3. Examination Stools

The weight scale should be durable and reasonably accurate (plus or minus 1 pound). A home-style bathroom scale is not recommended. Any medical supply house should be able to provide professional-quality scales in a variety of price ranges. Scale-mounted or wall-mounted devices to measure height are also easy to obtain.

A manual sphygmomanometer is recommended over an automatic version. The cuff on a manual sphygmomanometer is usually interchangeable, and the individual parts are more resistant to failure. The automatic instruments are one-size-fits-all and battery-dependent.

Stethoscopes come in all shapes, colors and sizes. Be sure to select one that has a diaphragm and a bell. A model with interchangeable parts is also a good idea. The smaller diaphragms and bells are useful when examining a child.

A high-quality electronic thermometer, which records temperature orally or from the ear canal, is recommended for evaluating the patient's temperature. Standard mercury models are also acceptable. However, they are not as time-efficient as their electronic counterparts. Temperature strips or patches that change color are not recommended. They are not as accurate as electronic thermometers or traditional mercury.

A variety of reflex hammers are acceptable. The traditional plexor, a reddish-orange rubber hammer with a triangular shape, is recommended. This hammer provides a pointed side for small tendons (biceps) and a broad, flat side for larger tendons (Achilles). The point at the bottom of the hammer handle is also useful for Babinski and sensory testing.

The examination table utilized will depend heavily on the doctor's choice of chiropractic techniques. The only universal requirement here is stability. The patient will be apprehensive during the exam if the table is unstable.

Inclinometers have replaced goniometers for measuring spinal range of motion. Manual inclinometer models are tedious and require calculations to determine the range of motion. Electronic models are less troublesome and capable of providing measurements without calculations, making them more time efficient.

THE PATIENT ATTIRE

The optimum attire for females is a patient gown. Males should disrobe to the waist and have bare feet. The primary reasons for disrobing are to allow accurate measurement of blood pressure and to check the Babinski response.

Secondarily, the suggested attire will increase the accuracy of weight measurement and provide easy transition to x-ray examination. A patient wearing a short-sleeved shirt need only remove socks and shoes for examination. Examiner discretion is always encouraged in matters of patient attire.

RECORDING THE EXAM

3. Positive results of orthopedic and neurological exam procedures should be recorded according to their intended meanings or interpretations.

4. Exam findings should be easy to record.

5. Exam results should be easy for third parties to read.

6. Exam procedures and the records of the procedures should protect the doctor/ practice should accusations of malpractice arise.

Frequently, clinicians record **any** response to a test as a positive or pathological finding. This is a habit that should be avoided. If the cervical compression test does not reproduce arm pain, it is negative. If the crossed straight leg raising (CSLR) test does not produce pain in the opposite extremity, it is negative. If both of these tests produce lower back pain for a patient during an exam, this result may be clinically significant, but it is not a positive or abnormal result for either test. Over-interpretation is misinterpretation and can lead to misdiagnosis and mistreatment. This is one of the primary reasons history and exam procedures that require interpretation should be performed by the doctor. Assistants and technicians may perform history and exam procedures that involve taking measurements (blood pressure, pulse, temperature, ROM) but not those that require interpretation.

Most practitioners are currently using examination forms that require check marks and circles, or computer programs that use a mouse or electronic pen. Handwritten notes are unusual these days. Convenient, easy-to-complete documents and programs are readily available. The problem seems to be in the consistency with which these tools are used. In the author's experience, all too often doctors subjected to peer review or malpractice situations have minimal or no exam findings recorded. The doctor often states that he or she was especially busy or running behind schedule at the time of the evaluation, and there was no time to record all the findings or that only positive findings were marked. True or not, remember the old saying, "If it isn't written down, it doesn't exist." Leaving the majority of an exam form unmarked is ill advised. The sample examination form provided in Appendix B allows the doctor to circle or check the majority of findings. Minimal writing is required and the form takes approximately two minutes to complete.

Once the results are recorded, anyone reviewing the records (other doctors, attorneys, insurance personnel or the patient) should be able to read the results. They may not be able to interpret or understand the meaning of a Nachlas test, for example, but they should be able to tell if it was positive or negative. Secret codes, unusual abbreviations and poor penmanship are to be avoided. A key should be provided to assist the reader if abbreviations are used.

Accurate records of good examination techniques are insurance polices against malpractice accusations. Haphazard clinical records and shoot-from-the-hip exams could be an Achilles heel for the doctor and the practice.

EXAM ORDER

Most exam forms are arranged by bodily region or by grouping all tests together for a particular pathology. These arrangements make the examination process tedious because patient positioning may change drastically between each test.

Once the content of an examination is selected, performance and efficiency are dependent upon the order of the individual components. It is best to arrange the tests first by patient position and then by the method of performance. For example, all tests requiring a patient to be seated should be completed prior to examining the patient in a standing position. All standing tests should be completed prior to examining the patient in a supine position, and so on. Tests which share similarities in body mechanics (slump, Bechterew's, Tripod) should be grouped together for performance. Following this same rationale, procedures that have been delegated to staff members/technicians (vital signs, etc.) should be grouped at the beginning of the exam. These procedures can be performed prior to the doctor's portion of the examination.

> **Practical Examination Strategy:**
>
> 7. A routine examination should be easy to perform and time efficient.

EXAMINATION SUMMARY
AND
FLOW CHART

The physical examination described in this text can be performed in 10 minutes or less. Obviously, initial attempts will take longer due to the learning curve associated with any new procedure or process. The algorithm of the examination process that appears on the following page will be helpful in refining the process for clinicians during their initial attempts to perform the examination.

Additionally, the sample examination form in Appendix B utilizes three different background shades in order to guide the examiner through the examination process.

1. Groups with **white** backgrounds are always performed in the order they appear on the examination form. These are the first sections to be performed and recorded when performing the examination.

2. Groups with **light gray** backgrounds represent observable, objective findings noted while performing the test groups with white backgrounds. These groups are the second sections to be recorded when completing the examination process.

3. Groups with **dark gray** backgrounds are for supplementary procedures. These sections may or may not be used during the examination process. If these groups of tests are performed, they are recorded last. If they are not utilized, a check mark or the initials of the examiner should be recorded in the space provided prior to the statement, "Use of this section not indicated."

Thus Groups 1, 4, 5, 6, 7, 11, 13, 14 and 15 are performed consecutively. Results for Groups 2, 3, 8 and 12 are based solely on observations made while performing Groups 1, 4, 5, 6, 7, 11, 13, 14 and 15. Groups 9, 10 and 17 and/or 16 and 17 are used for further evaluation, confirming results or ruling out malingering.

Examination Flow Chart

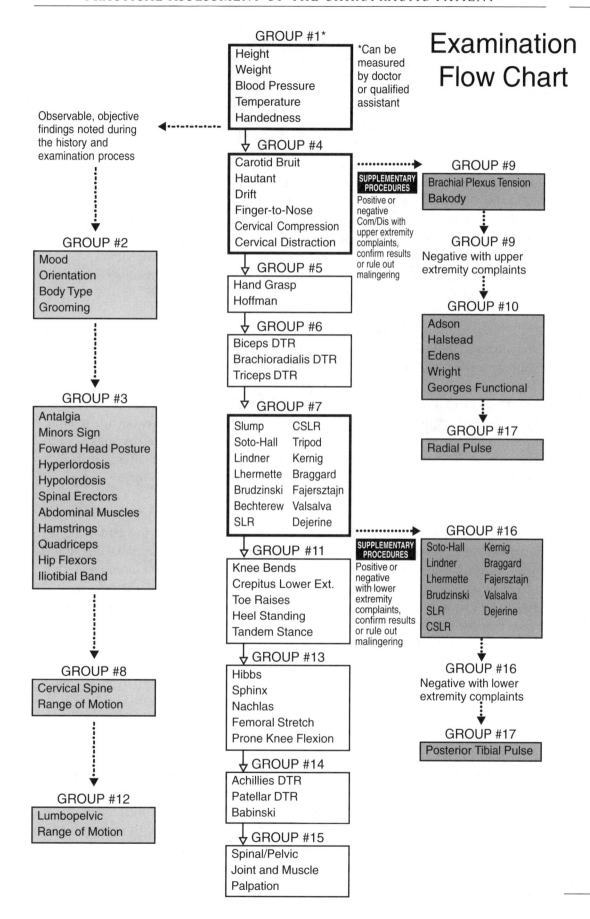

GROUP #1*

- Height
- Weight
- Blood Pressure
- Temperature
- Handedness

*Can be measured by doctor or qualified assistant

Observable, objective findings noted during the history and examination process

GROUP #2

- Mood
- Orientation
- Body Type
- Grooming

GROUP #3

- Antalgia
- Minors Sign
- Foward Head Posture
- Hyperlordosis
- Hypolordosis
- Spinal Erectors
- Abdominal Muscles
- Hamstrings
- Quadriceps
- Hip Flexors
- Iliotibial Band

GROUP #8

- Cervical Spine
- Range of Motion

GROUP #12

- Lumbopelvic
- Range of Motion

GROUP #4

- Carotid Bruit
- Hautant
- Drift
- Finger-to-Nose
- Cervical Compression
- Cervical Distraction

SUPPLEMENTARY PROCEDURES
Positive or negative Com/Dis with upper extremity complaints, confirm results or rule out malingering

GROUP #5

- Hand Grasp
- Hoffman

GROUP #6

- Biceps DTR
- Brachioradialis DTR
- Triceps DTR

GROUP #7

Slump	CSLR
Soto-Hall	Tripod
Lindner	Kernig
Lhermette	Braggard
Brudzinski	Fajersztajn
Bechterew	Valsalva
SLR	Dejerine

GROUP #11

- Knee Bends
- Crepitus Lower Ext.
- Toe Raises
- Heel Standing
- Tandem Stance

SUPPLEMENTARY PROCEDURES
Positive or negative with lower extremity complaints, confirm results or rule out malingering

GROUP #13

- Hibbs
- Sphinx
- Nachlas
- Femoral Stretch
- Prone Knee Flexion

GROUP #14

- Achillies DTR
- Patellar DTR
- Babinski

GROUP #15

- Spinal/Pelvic
- Joint and Muscle
- Palpation

GROUP #9

- Brachial Plexus Tension
- Bakody

GROUP #9
Negative with upper extremity complaints

GROUP #10

- Adson
- Halstead
- Edens
- Wright
- Georges Functional

GROUP #17

- Radial Pulse

GROUP #16

Soto-Hall	Kernig
Lindner	Braggard
Lhermette	Fajersztajn
Brudzinski	Valsalva
SLR	Dejerine
CSLR	

GROUP #16
Negative with lower extremity complaints

GROUP #17

- Posterior Tibial Pulse

13

TEST SELECTION

Practical Examination Strategy:

8. Exam procedures should not be limited to tests related solely to a specific chiropractic technique.

If a patient is receiving chiropractic adjustments, the patient is presumed to be subluxated. This indicates that tests for subluxation based on the doctor's choice of techniques are among the most important performed. Some may say these are the only tests necessary. Despite an emphasis on the subluxation complex, doctors of chiropractic are not excused from the responsibility of ruling out other disease processes or contraindications to adjustments. (Nor are doctors excused for abandoning skills learned in school or failing to stay abreast of professional advancements.)

Tests specific to any single chiropractic technique are not incorporated into the Practical Exam Process. The Practical Exam can be used prior to, or in conjunction with any chiropractic technique exam.

Doctors who treat only the spinal areas of chief complaint and full-spine practitioners both can benefit from the examination procedures recommended here. Doctors treating localized spinal areas can use the tests to rule out involvement of other regions prior to beginning care. Full-spine practitioners have the advantage of testing all regions that will receive treatment. In either situation, the exam will apply to the majority of patients with spinal/pelvic complaints.

Practical Examination Strategies:

9. Exam procedures in chiropractic practice should be applicable to patients with a variety of complaints related to the head, spine, pelvis and extremities.

10. The procedures utilized during examination should be well-accepted and widely used.

The use of examination techniques learned at accredited institutions and used by both the medical and chiropractic professions is a good practice. There is minimal doubt as to the interpretation and significance of these procedures. Relying upon examination techniques obtained from unaccredited institutions or used by an isolated group of practitioners is risky. This is not to say that such procedures are without merit. It only means that the interpretation and significance of the procedures may not be widely known or accepted. Obscure procedures present a problem when the clinician must confirm a diagnosis, justify a course of treatment or defend an accusation of malpractice. Procedures that may be considered obscure should be accompanied by an examination containing more widely accepted procedures.

It is probable that every patient who enters a chiropractic office is subluxated, yet not every patient needs an adjustment. Patients with primary cancers, secondary cancers, aortic aneurysms, carotid artery blockage, vertebral artery compromise, cauda equina syndrome, meningitis, upper motor neuron lesions and other ominous conditions may be better off in the hands of our allopathic medical colleagues. Some doctors say, "I don't treat the disease, only the subluxations." True, but think about this carefully! The benefits of any type of treatment should outweigh the risks. Remember the rule of the golden hammer: "When your only tool is a hammer, everything looks like a nail." Don't fall into this mindset.

It is difficult, if not impossible, to rely solely on orthopedic and neurological tests to identify ominous conditions, because some are neither specific nor sensitive. Still, most physical, orthopedic and neurological exam procedures are noninvasive, easy to perform and cost effective.

Some tests that are neither sensitive nor specific have become traditional (George's and other vascular tests). This is often due to a lack of more reliable tests. One may argue against the use of such tests, feeling they are pointless or a waste of time. After all, if tests with low specificity and sensitivity were invasive and/or expensive, it would be difficult to qualify them as necessary for chiropractic or medical purposes. Discontinuing use of these tests is not a problem until accusations of malpractice arise. If the tests are traditionally used, the plaintiff can easily find someone who will swear that, in their expert opinion, not performing the tests was a breach of the standard of care. It is recommended that tests that have become traditional and can provide even a remote degree of protection for the patient and the doctor be continued as long as they are not invasive or expensive.

Practical Examination Strategy:

11. Exam techniques should seek to identify or rule out ominous conditions and contraindications to chiropractic adjustment.

THE EXAM

Group One Tests

1. Height
2. Weight
3. Blood Pressure
4. Temperature
5. Handedness

Physicians Current Procedural Terminology Coding Manuals provide a list of required elements for examining a patient (See Table 4). Each exam level mandates the performance of a specific number of these elements. The content of the examination should meet the requirements for the CPT billing code listed for the exam.

TABLE 4

Exam Requirements for CPT codes 99201-99205	
Code	**Number of Elements**
99201	One to five elements identified by bullets
99202	At least six elements identified by a bullet
99203	At least 12 elements identified by a bullet
99204/99205	All elements identified by a bullet

Adapted from E/M Coding Made Easy, 3rd Edition, by: PMIC

Doctors should cross-reference all exams with CPT code descriptions (See Tables 4, 5 and 6). It is very easy for utilization reviewers to downgrade an exam code to a lower level due to inadequate documentation. If an exam does not meet the requirements for the CPT code submitted, the insurance carrier accuses the doctor of "up coding" or charging for a higher-level procedure than was actually performed. This reflects poorly on the doctor and the profession and may result in penalties.

TABLE 5

ELEMENTS OF MUSCULOSKELETAL EXAMINATIONS

Constitutional
- Measurement of **any three of the following seven** vital signs: 1) sitting or standing blood pressure; 2) supine blood pressure; 3) pulse rate and regularity; 4) respiration; 5) temperature; 6) height; and 7) weight (May be measured and recorded by ancillary staff.)
- General appearance of patient (e.g., development, nutrition, body habitus, deformities, attention to grooming)

Cardiovascular
- Examination of peripheral vascular system by observation (e.g., swelling, varicosities) and palpation (e.g., pulses, temperature, edema, tenderness)

Lymphatic
- Palpation of lymph nodes in neck, axilla, groin and/or other locations.

Musculoskeletal
- Examination of gait and station

Examination of joint(s), bone(s) and muscle(s)/tendon(s) of **four of the following six** areas: 1) head and neck; 2) spine, ribs and pelvis; 3) right upper extremity; 4) left upper extremity; 5) right lower extremity; and 6) left lower extremity. The examination of a given area includes:

- Inspection, percussion and/or palpation with notation of any misalignment, asymmetry, crepitation, defects, tenderness, masses or effusions
- Assessment of range of motion with notation of any pain (e.g., straight leg raising), crepitation or contracture
- Assessment of stability with notation of any dislocation (luxation), subluxation or laxity
- Assessment of muscle strength and tone (e.g., flaccid, cogwheel, spastic) with notation of any atrophy or abnormal movements

Note: For the comprehensive level of examination, all four of the elements identified by a bullet must be performed and documented for each of four anatomic areas. For the three lower levels of examination, each element is counted separately for each body area. For example, assessing range of motion in two extremities constitutes two elements.

Skin
- Inspection and/or palpation of skin and subcutaneous tissue (e.g., scars, rashes, lesions, Café-au-lait spots, ulcers) in **four of the following six** areas: 1) head and neck; 2) trunk; 3) right upper extremity; 4) left upper extremity; 5) right lower extremity; and 6) left lower extremity

Note: For the comprehensive level, the examination of all four anatomic areas must be performed and documented. For the three lower levels of examination, each body area is counted separately. For example, inspection and/or palpation of the skin and subcutaneous tissue of two extremities constitutes two elements.

Neurological/ Psychiatric
- Test coordination (e.g., finger/nose, heel/knee/shin, rapid alternating movements in the upper and lower extremities, evaluation of fine motor coordination in young children)
- Examination of deep tendon reflexes and/or nerve stretch test with notation of pathological reflexes (e.g., Babinski)
- Examination of sensation (e.g., by touch, pin, vibration, proprioception)

Brief assessment of mental status including:
- Orientation to time, place and person
- Mood and effect (e.g., depression, anxiety, agitation)

Adapted from E/M Coding Made Easy, 3rd Edition, by: PMIC

TABLE 6

ELEMENTS OF NEUROLOGICAL EXAMINATION	
Constitutional	• Measurement of **any three of the following seven** vital signs: 1) sitting or standing blood pressure; 2) supine blood pressure; 3) pulse rate and regularity; 4) respiration; 5) temperature; 6) height; and 7) weight (May be measured and recorded by ancillary staff.) • General appearance of patient (e.g., development, nutrition, body habitus, deformities, attention to grooming)
Head and Face/ Eyes	• Ophthalmoscopic examination of optic discs (e.g., size, C/D ratio, appearance) and posterior segments (e.g., vessel changes, exudates, hemorrhages)
Cardiovascular	• Examination of carotid arteries (e.g., pulse amplitude, bruits) • Auscultation of heart with notation of abnormal sounds and murmurs • Examination of peripheral vascular system by observation (e.g., swelling, varicosities) and palpation (e.g., pulses, temperature, edema, tenderness)
Musculoskeletal	• Examination of gait and station Assessment of motor function including: • Muscle strength in upper and lower extremities • Muscle tone in upper and lower extremities (e.g., flaccid, cogwheel, spastic) with notation of any atrophy or abnormal movements (e.g., fasciculation, tardive dyskinesia)
Extremities/ Skin	*(See Musculoskeletal)*
Neurological	Evaluation of higher integrative function including: • Orientation to time, place and person • Recent and remote memory • Attention span and concentration • Language (e.g., naming objects, repeating phrases, spontaneous speech) • Fund of knowledge (e.g., awareness of current events, past history, vocabulary) Test the following cranial nerves: • 2nd cranial nerve (e.g., visual acuity, visual fields, fundi) • 3rd, 4th and 6th cranial nerves (e.g., pupils, eye movements) • 5th cranial nerve (e.g., facial sensation, corneal reflexes) • 7th cranial nerve (e.g., facial symmetry, strength) • 8th cranial nerve (e.g., hearing with tuning fork, whispered voice and/or finger rub) • 9th cranial nerve (e.g., spontaneous or reflex palate movement) • 11th cranial nerve (e.g., shoulder shrug strength) • 12th cranial nerve (e.g., tongue protrusion) • Examination of sensation (e.g., by touch, pin, vibration, proprioception) • Examination of deep tendon reflexes in upper and lower extremities with notation of pathological reflexes (e.g., Babinski) • Test coordination (e.g., finger/nose, heel/knee/shin, rapid alternating movements in the upper and lower extremities, evaluation of fine motor coordination in young children)

Adapted from E/M Coding Made Easy, 3rd Edition, by: PMIC

This examination includes 14 bullets from the required elements for new or established patient exams (See Table 7). When combined with an appropriate history, the procedures recommended in the text are appropriately coded as a 99203-level examination for new patients and a 99214-level examination for established patients. Both of these examination levels require 12 elements (See Table 1). The examination is designed to be performed in 10 minutes. The remainder of the time elements for codes 99203 and 99214 (15 to 20 minutes) are met during the history and decision-making processes.

TABLE 7

ORTHOPEDIC AND NEUROLOGICAL BULLETS FOR PRACTICAL ASSESSMENT OF THE CHIROPRACTIC PATIENT
Constitutional   • Vital signs: height, weight, blood pressure, temperature   • General appearance: body type, grooming
Cardiovascular   • Carotid Arteries: auscultation of carotid arteries   • Pulses: palpation of radial and post tibial pulses
Musculoskeletal   • Gait and station: observation of antalgic posture or gait, all items in group 3   • Palpation: spine and pelvis   • Range of motion: full spine, lower extremities (knee bends)   • Stability: palpation, orthopedic tests   • Muscle strength: drift, hand grasp, knee bends, heel walk, toe raises
Neurological   • Muscle tone in upper and lower extremities (cog wheel, flacid, spasm, atrophy, fasciculations)   • Coordination: finger to nose, tandem stance   • Deep tendon reflexes: biceps, brachioradialis, triceps, patella, Achilles, Pathological reflexes: Hoffman, Babinski   • Orientation: person, place, time   • Mood: pleasant, calm, depressed, anxious, agitated

Even with the inclusion of additional orthopedic and neurological tests, the exam cannot be upgraded to a higher level without the inclusion of all elements identified by bullets in the CPT coding manual. Tests specific to chiropractic techniques are not included in the exam elements in the CPT Manual. Thus, they will not count.

The first elements listed for CPT coding are constitutional elements consisting of general appearance and vital signs. Use of these elements is standard procedure for medical practice but not chiropractic practice. This is unfortunate because these exams provide valuable information about the patient's general health or constitution.

Seven vital signs are listed by the *ChiroCode DeskBook, CPT Procedures*: Sitting or standing blood pressure; supine blood pressure; pulse rate and regularity; respiration; temperature; height; and weight. At least three of these signs should be measured in order to meet the requirements for this element.

The medical profession relies upon pulse, respiration and blood pressure as baseline indicators of a patient's health.[3] The triad of temperature, weight and height also plays a vital role as a baseline indicator of general health.

Height, weight, blood pressure and temperature were included in the Practical Examination to meet the requirement of recording vital signs and because they should have the greatest effect on diagnosing (and differential diagnosing) neuromusculoskeletal conditions treated in chiropractic practice.

The height of the patient is important when compared to the weight of the patient. Excess weight on an individual with a small frame could be considered a cause of (or a complicating factor for) lower back complaints. Stress on the joints of the lower extremities is also a concern.

Third parties reviewing a patient's records are provided a mental image of the patient by these measurements. This is important in today's era of utilization review because there seems to be a misconception by many utilization reviewers that all patients are healthy specimens with physiques of Olympic stature.

Beyond its relationship to height, body weight plays an important role in determining x-ray settings and ordering MR scans. Larger patients are often easier to radiograph on an x-ray table as compared to a standing buckey. Patients who exceed 300 pounds will not fit into the gantry of many conventional MR units. An open unit is required for these individuals.

Once height and weight are recorded, the patient is instructed to sit on the examination table. The patient will remain in this position for several series of tests.

The purpose of orthopedic and neurologic testing is to reproduce the patient's chief complaint. Because the patient may report an exacerbation of symptoms just after examination,[1] it is a good idea to tell the patient prior to the exam that symptoms may increase. This dispels any thoughts that the doctor made the condition worse or otherwise caused harm during the exam. To help reduce post-exam pain, perform maneuvers with multiple implications only once and record the results according to the patient's response. For example, cervical flexion is the primary maneuver for Soto Hall, Lindner and Lhermette tests. The cervical spine should be flexed once and the patient's response recorded. Unless the patient's response was vague or uncertain, the examiner should avoid flexing the cervical spine repeatedly for each individual test. Performing tests that share a particular patient position (i.e., sitting, standing, prone) and movement (flexion, extension) as a group enhances efficiency and minimizes patient distress.

Practical Examination Strategy:

12. Exams should minimize discomfort for the patient.

Doctors of chiropractic are frequently the only doctors patients will see on a routine basis. This places the chiropractor in the role of the primary care provider. Since hypertension is a risk factor for cardiovascular events and is usually asymptomatic, establishing a baseline blood pressure for new patients and periodic screening thereafter is a good idea. Cardiovascular conditions are of primary concern in chiropractic practice, especially strokes and aortic aneurysms.

George's Cardiovascular Craniocervical Functional Tests include a bilateral blood pressure measurement. A difference of 10 millimeters of mercury between the left and right sides is said to be an indication of subclavian artery stenosis or occlusion on the side with the lower pressure.[4] Upper extremity pressure differences can also be a result of supravalvular aortic stenosis.[5] Additional information on George's test is provided later under test Groups Four and Ten.

Bilateral measurement of blood pressure will not always be necessary or possible. Patients with an unremarkable cardiovascular history and a normal first reading may not require a second measurement. Patients who have had a breast removed should not have blood pressure measurements performed in the upper extremity on the side of the removal. If both breasts have been removed, blood pressure should be recorded in the lower extremities. A similar situation exists for dialysis patients who have a shunt or stint implanted in an extremity. Do not compress a shunt or stint with a blood pressure cuff.

Temperature is usually elevated when the body is fighting an infection. While the number of infectious processes are too numerous to list, a few warrant mention because they frequently cause symptoms that may result in a patient seeking chiropractic care.

Kidney infections can cause lower back pain. Lung infections can cause thoracic spine pain. Meningitis can cause neck and head pain. Other infections in the head and neck can cause neck stiffness secondary to lymph node swelling. Routine temperature measurement aids in the differential diagnosis of these conditions.

Fig. 4A, B, C, D. Examples of Pseudo-ambidexterity

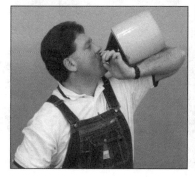
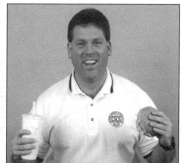
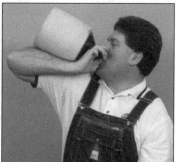

Handedness is not a constitutional sign. However, it is an important bit of information in the evaluation of a chiropractic patient and is ascertained by simply asking the patient if he is right or left handed. If the patient relates that he is ambidextrous, further questioning may be necessary to determine the extent of the patient's ambidextrous abilities. Some individuals say they are ambidextrous simply because they can use a fork or drink with either hand. This is pseudoambidexterity (Fig. 4: A-D). A more realistic version of ambidexterity would be a person capable of writing or throwing a ball with either hand.

Handedness is important to determine in musculoskeletal evaluation for four reasons. Grip strength is the first reason. The dominant hand is typically 5 to 10 percent stronger than the non-dominant hand.[1] This should be remembered if the hand grasp test described later in this text indicates a need for grip strength testing using a dynamometer. If dynamometer testing shows grip strength to be equal, the patient is truly ambidextrous, uses the non-dominant hand more than the average person or has a 5 to 10 percent loss of strength in the dominant hand. If the dominant hand is weaker than the non-dominant hand, the percentage of loss must include the 5 to 10 percent of additional strength normally present in the dominant hand.

Impairment rating is the second reason for the importance of determining handedness. The final rating for a patient with upper extremity impairment is usually not assigned until the side of handedness is considered.

When a final figure is reached for an impaired upper extremity, the impairment is reduced for the non-dominant hand prior to conversion to a whole-person figure. The upper extremity value is reduced by 5 percent if the extremity value is 5 to 50 percent or by 10 percent if the extremity value is 51 to 100 percent. The final upper extremity value for a dominant hand is not altered prior to conversion to a whole-person figure.[6] Please note that the rule of preferred vs. non-preferred hand may be regulated by state law.[6]

The use of side posture manipulation for the lumbar spine is the third reason for determining handedness. Medical researcher H.F. Farfan has written extensively on the scientific basis for manipulation. One of his theories relates to injuries of the alternating layers of fibers that make up the annulus of an intervertebral disc. The annulus is composed of multiple layers, or laminations, of obliquely oriented fibers. Each layer runs in the opposite direction of the adjoining layer. The orientation of alternating layers helps the disc withstand torsion (twisting) to the right and left.

In theory, a person stresses fibers that resist torsion to one side more than the other due to the use of a preferred extremity.[7] A right-handed individual always twists to the left when throwing a ball or swinging a bat, racquet or club. This places the majority of stress on the annular fibers that resist left rotation and minimal stress on the fibers that resist right

Fig. 5A. Right Farfan's Torsion Test

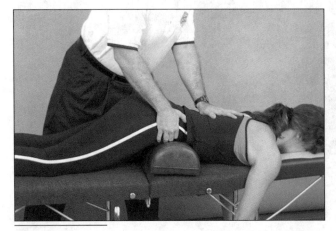

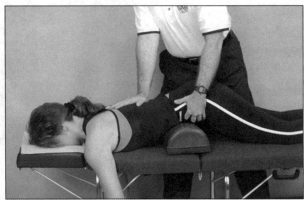

Fig. 5B. Left Farfan's Torsion Test

rotation. This repeated stress to one side produces what Farfan terms a torsion injury.

Farfan's torsion test seeks to identify patients with lumbar torsion injuries. The test is classified by the side of the hemipelvis lifted during the test.[8] The test is performed by stabilizing the lumbar spine of a patient in a prone position, with the lumbar lordosis reduced, and then lifting the hemipelvis (Fig. 5: A–B). The test is then repeated on the opposite side. Lifting the right hemipelvis simulates left rotation; lifting the left hemipelvis simulates right rotation. Reproduction of the patient's lower back pain is a positive finding. A right-handed individual repeatedly twisting to the left will create a left torsion injury, which could produce a positive right Farfan's torsion test. A left-handed individual repeatedly twisting to the right will create a right torsion injury, which will produce a positive left Farfan's torsion test. A right-handed patient with a left torsion injury should receive side posture manipulation with the right side up while a left-handed individual with a right torsion injury should receive side posture manipulation with the left side up. *In short, side posture manipulation would typically be performed with the patient's side of handedness up.* Side posture manipulation may be contraindicated for patients exhibiting both left and right torsion injuries.

Brain electrical activity mapping, or BEAM, is the last reason for determining handedness. BEAM testing correlates the results from electroencephalogram testing, brain stem auditory evoked responses, visual evoked responses and a cognitive test in order to identify occult brain injuries. The data obtained from the four tests is fed into a computer, which compares it to a database based on age, sex and *handedness.*[9] BEAM testing is not a routine evaluation in chiropractic practice. However, doctors of chiropractic should be familiar with the availability of the test when dealing with whiplash and post-concussion syndromes.

Measurement of vital signs and handedness can be delegated to support staff for completion prior to the doctor's portion of the examination. These tests are measurements that do not require interpretation at the time they are recorded.

Group Two Tests

1. Mood
2. Orientation
3. Body Type
4. Grooming

Evaluation of the patient's constitution continues beyond vital signs with observations of mood, orientation (person, place and time), body type and grooming. These observations provide insight in three critical areas. First, they assist in meeting CPT coding requirements. Second, they paint a picture of the patient for third parties reviewing the exam results. Third, they can provide objective evidence of improvement. In all cases information is obtained without the performance of physical maneuvers.

Mood, body type and grooming fall under the general-appearance element of the patient's constitution. Orientations to person, place and time fall under the neurological element for brief assessment of mental status (Tables 5 and 6). Thus, two required elements are covered by mood, orientation, body type and grooming. Three required elements are satisfied to this point in the exam with height, weight, blood pressure and temperature having already been performed.

CPT coding is stressed here to emphasize the importance of including the initial procedures described. Chiropractic examinations cannot meet higher-level coding requirements without this first series of tests.

The patient's mood can paint a variety of pictures. Pleasant, calm patients are generally cooperative. Depressed patients may be victims of chronic pain. Anxious patients are often uncomfortable with their surroundings (first visit to a new doctor) and/or they are experiencing significant pain. Patients who have been badgered by friends and family to see a doctor or forced to submit to an independent medical evaluation may be agitated.

Orientation to person, place and time is usually easy to observe from the manner in which the patient completes entrance forms and/or participates in the history process. The patient who does not recognize himself or others is not oriented to person. A patient who dates a form "1994" today is not oriented to time. A patient who asks for an insurance quote for his automobile during the history process is not oriented to place.

Body type has a direct relationship to height and weight measurements recorded earlier. Ectomorphs are slender and tall. Endomorphs are round or pear-shaped. Mesomorphs are narrow-wasted, broad-shouldered and muscular.[10] The terms athletic, asthenic and pyknic have been used for mesomorphic, ectomorphic and endomorphic, respectively.[1]

Patients experiencing significant pain often appear poorly groomed. Patients with shoulder problems may have difficulty washing or combing their hair. Patients with lower back problems may have trouble putting on socks/shoes and may wear bedroom slippers to the doctor's office.

Bathing may be infrequent during bouts of severe pain for many patients. Objective evidence of patient improvement can be seen when a patient who was initially anxious, unbathed and wearing a bathrobe and slippers returns to the office pleasant, clean and neatly dressed.

Grooming can also provide indirect evidence of patient compliance. The patient who does not bathe regularly and gives little attention to personal appearance is not likely to follow through with home therapies and exercise. Conversely, the patient who routinely makes an effort to look his best may have the self-discipline needed to follow home care programs.

Observation of these factors can coincide with the history and examination process. If the doctor conducts the problem-focused history, these elements can be recorded as the exam begins. If the problem-focused history is performed by support staff, the doctor should record observations after the examination is complete.

Group Three Tests

1. Observation for Antalgia
2. Minors Sign
3. Forward Head Posture
4. Lumbar Hyperlordosis
5. Lumbar Hypolordosis
6. Hamstring Tension
7. Quadriceps Tension
8. Hip Flexor Tension
9. Iliotibial Band Tension
10. Spinal Erectors
11. Abdominal Muscles

Recording the presence or absence of antalgic posturing is an exam procedure that relies solely on observation. Items in Group Three fall under the CPT element of musculoskel-etal inspection, the fourth element to be included in the examination. The remaining elements covered in the complete examination process are listed in Table 7.

Subluxations can cause multiple forms of antalgia. Head and cervical-spine antalgia are usually present in torticollis. Thoracic antalgia may be seen after a compression frac-ture. Lumbar and pelvic antalgia can be the result of disc herniation, spasm or lumbopelvic sprain. A patient with an abducted upper extremity may have an acute radiculitis. A painful lower extremity is usually revealed by an antalgic gait.

Fig. 6.
Minors Sign

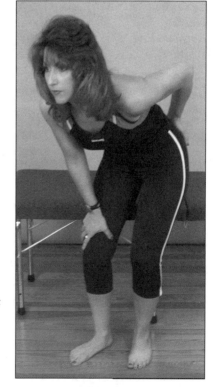

Minors sign is an observable orthopedic sign commonly seen in patients with sacroiliac joint dysfunctions, abnormal lumbopelvic rhythm, sciatic radiculitis, lumbosacral strains/sprains and disc syndromes. The author has found this to be one of the most common signs of SI joint fixation. The tests may also indicate dystrophies or myotonia. The sign is exhibited when a patient moves from a seated to a standing position. The symptomatic patient balances his weight on the unaffected side while holding his back and flexing the hip and knee on the affected side while rising[11] (Fig. 6).

Minors sign may be observed at several different points during the examination. Observation of the sign may be made by the doctor or staff when the patient rises to move from the reception room to the examination room or when the patient moves from a seated to a stand-ing position during the exam process. There is usually no need to ask the patient to perform the procedure separately.

In addition to demonstrating Minors sign during the examination process, the patient may also describe a positive Minors sign during the history. When asked what factors re-create or aggravate the symptoms, the patient will often state that getting up from a chair and the first several steps after are the most painful movements. The patient will report diminished pain after the first several steps.

Notation of a forward head posture is very important during the course of musculoskeletal exam. Multiple musculoskeletal dysfunctions, compression syndromes, peripheral nerve entrapments and vascular dysfunctions can occur from a forward head position resulting in local and/or referred pain in the body's upper quadrant. The effects of head positioning are far-reaching as the body will always adjust itself under the head.[12]

Forward displacement is determined by comparing the head position to its normal center of gravity. The head's center of gravity is at a point just anterior to the cervical spine and just superior to the tempromandibular joint (Fig. 7: A–B). Forward displacement by even an inch is significant. It is recommended that the reader obtain further information regarding forward head syndromes by reading Thomas F. Shaw's contribution to John Mennell's book, *The Musculoskeletal System, Differential Diagnosis from Symptoms and Physical Signs* (Aspen Publishers).

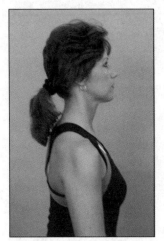

*Fig. 7A.
Normal Head
Position*

The degree of the patient's lumbar lordosis and tone/tension of the hamstring, gluteal, spinal erector, hip flexor and abdominal muscles are all closely linked. The assessment of individuals prior to implementation of resistance training (weight training) considers the link between these structures.[10] Two posture types are identified that may cause complications or result in injury during training. The first is the individual with hypolordosis. Hypolordosis may indicate tight hamstring and gluteal muscles or weak spinal erector muscles (Remember, hypolordosis may also be due to antalgic posture). Correcting these postural disturbances prior to beginning weight training is thought to reduce the risk of training injuries. Correction involves stretching the hamstring and gluteal muscles while strengthening the spinal erectors.

The second type is the individual with hyperlordosis. Hyperlordosis may indicate tight hip flexor and spinal erector muscles or weak, elongated abdominal muscles. Correcting these postural distortions prior to beginning weight training is again thought to reduce the risk of training injuries. Correction involves stretching the hip flexor and spinal erector muscles and strengthening the abdominal muscles.[10]

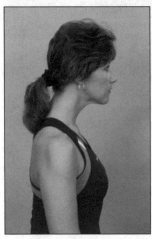

*Fig. 7B.
Forward
Displacement
of the Head*

The author has found the postural distortions above to be helpful in intitial screening of asymptomatic individuals to identify those who may eventually develop lumbopelvic problems. This is important, as most radiographic findings have not proven to be pathognomonic,[13] and orthopedic/neurological tests performed on asymptomatic individuals are often unfruitful. Lumbar hyper or hypolordosis is easily observed during the course of the examination.

While radiographic information alone may not be completely diagnostic, clinical observations of head placement and lordosis can be compared to lateral spinal radiographs to confirm results. A variety of measurements exist for lateral cervical and lumbar radiographs meant to assist in the determination of centers of gravity and degrees of lordosis.[14]

Tight hamstrings may be noted during the slump test in Group Seven. Tripod sign may occur because of tight hamstrings (Fig. 8: A). The same holds true of straight leg raising testing in the supine position – there is more on these tests later. Occasionally the shins of a patient in the prone position will not rest on the footrest of an adjusting table. This is an indication of tight hamstring muscles. In these cases the knees appear to be fixed in 5 to 10 degrees of flexion (Fig. 8: B). This phenomenon can occur unilaterally.

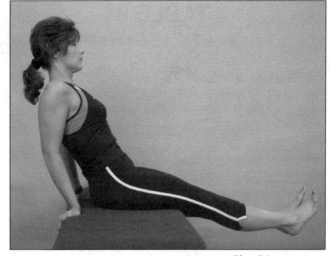

Fig. 8A.
Tripod Sign

Tight quadriceps can be noted during deep knee bends in Group Eleven and/or Nachlas, femoral stretch and prone knee flexion tests in Group Thirteen. Tight quadriceps may produce repeated crepitus in the knee joint during deep knee bends. This will need to be differentiated from other types of knee joint crepitus. Nachlas, femoral stretch and prone knee flexion tests all involve flexing the knee to approximate the patient's heel to the buttocks. The heel will usually touch the buttocks in a normal subject. Patients with tight quadriceps will report a tight/pulling feeling or the heel will not touch the buttocks (Fig. 9: A–B). Tight quadriceps will also have to be differentiated from positive findings for Nachlas, femoral stretch and prone knee flexion tests. Differences are described under Group Thirteen and in Table 8.

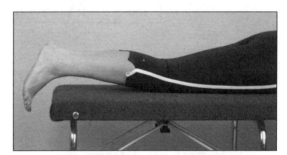

Fig. 8B.
Failure of the knee to fully extend in a prone position due to tight hamstring muscles.

Tight hip flexors can also be identified during the performance of Nachlas, femoral stretch and prone knee flexion testing. Approximating the heel to the buttocks during these tests may result in spontaneous flexion of the

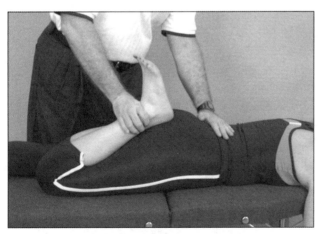

Fig. 9A. Normal (heel to buttocks).

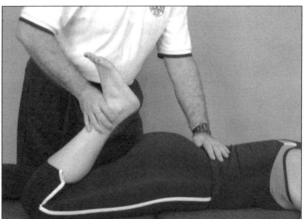

Fig. 9B. Failure of heel to meet buttocks due to tight quadriceps muscles.

27

TABLE 8

Interpretation of Patient Responses to Group Thirteen	
Location of Symptom	**Meaning**
Pain in the cervical region	Cervical facet syndrome
Lower back pain	Positive Sphinx
Pain at the lumbosacral junction	Positive Nachlas
Pain in either SI joint	Positive Nachlas
Pulling/stretching sensation in the anterior thigh	Tight quadriceps muscles
Pain or paresthesia in the anterior thigh along the course of the femoral nerve	Positive femoral stretch test
Post-testing loss or decrease in reflex and/or motor function in the home leg	Positive prone knee flexion test

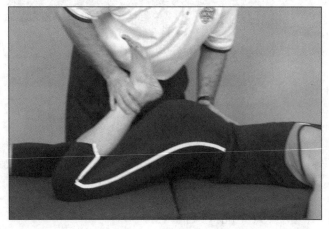

Fig. 10. Positive Ely's Test: Tight hip flexors, rectus femoris and/or psoas muscle.

ipsilateral hip. Some resources list the rectus femoris as the muscle primarily responsible for hip flexion.[1] Others list the psoas as the culprit.[8] Spontaneous hip flexion in response to knee flexion is a positive Ely's test (Fig. 10).

Repeated crepitus during knee bends performed in Group Eleven may indicate tension in the iliotibial band. Snapping will be felt or heard over the greater trochanter or the lateral aspect of the knee. Tension in the iliotibial band can lead to tendonitis/bursitis in either location. Tension in the iliotibial band is often associated with SI joint dysfunction.

Obers and Nobel's tests will help confirm the origin of crepitus noted in the iliotibial band during knee bends. The reader is referred to McGee[1] for additional information.

A direct test of the spinal erectors is not performed. Their condition is inferred by the degree of the patient's lordosis. As stated earlier, patients with hypolordosis typically have weak spinal erector muscles, and patients with hyperlordosis typically have tight spinal erector muscles.

The condition of the patient's abdominal musculature can easily be assessed by observation. Confirmation of the condition of the abdominal muscles can be ascertained by palpation or by having the patient perform crunches or sit-ups. Having the patient perform a crunch and then hold the crunched position isometrically works well. The longer the patient can sustain the position, the stronger the abdominal muscles.

Group Four Tests

1. Carotid Auscultation
2. Drift
3. Hautant
4. Finger-to-Nose
5. Cervical Compression
6. Cervical Distraction

Auscultation of the carotid arteries is a standard neurological procedure and a part of George's test.[4,15] Auscultation is performed by placing the bell of the stethoscope over the carotid artery just anterior and medial to the sternocleido-mastoid muscle (Fig. 11). The bell is preferred over the diaphragm of the stethoscope because low-pitched sounds are easier to hear with the bell.

The patient is instructed to stop breathing to prevent breathing sounds from masking vascular sounds. Auscultating for a few seconds prior to instructing the patient to stop breathing will provide a sharp contrast between breaths and other sounds.

With the exception of benign venous hums, blood flow is normally silent. Bruits are murmurs that suggest vascular turbulence. They may be present with aneurysms, occlusive vascular disease and vascular malformations. In patients with coronary artery disease, hypertension and diabetes, bruits indicate a risk of stroke.

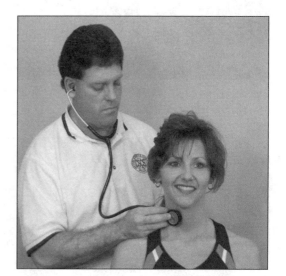

*Fig. 11.
Auscultation
of the
carotid artery.*

Narrowing of the vessel must be 50 percent before a bruit is audible. Occlusion beyond 50 percent is associated with an increase in loudness. Bruits disappear when an occlusion reaches 95 percent or greater.[15] Thus, the absence of a bruit does not rule out pathology. Correlation of findings must be made with the patient's history and other cardiovascular findings. The presence of a bruit indicates a need for additional evaluation by Doppler ultrasonography, angiography, MR scan or CT scan.

Identifying motor dysfunction originating in the cerebrum or brain stem is accomplished by testing for drift of the upper and/or lower extremities. Upper extremity drift is tested with the patient seated. The patient extends his arms anteriorly with the hands supinated. The patient is instructed to close his eyes and hold this position for 15 to 30 seconds (Fig. 12). The arms will remain supinated and parallel to the floor in unaffected individuals. The arm will pronate and drop (drift from position) on the affected side in individuals with weakness (Fig. 13).

Lower extremity drift is tested with the patient prone. The knees should be bent at 90 degrees and the lower legs should be vertical (Fig. 14). The patient's eyes should be

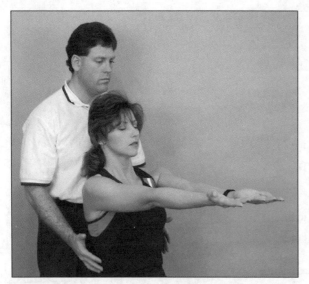

Fig. 12. Upper Extremity Drift Test: starting/normal position.

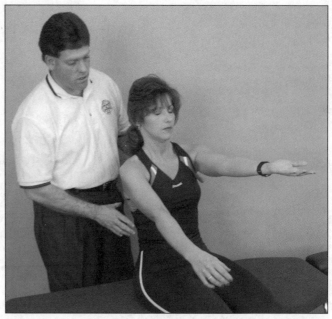

Fig. 13. Positive Drift Test: upper extremities.

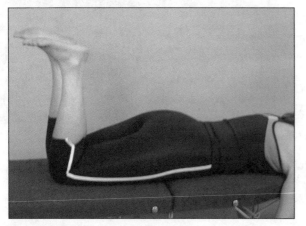

Fig. 14. Lower Extremity Drift Test: starting/normal position.

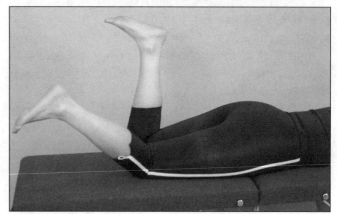

Fig. 15. Positive Drift Test: lower extremities.

closed. This position is also held for 15 to 30 seconds. A positive finding is dropping (drifting) of the leg on the affected side (Fig. 15). It is generally not necessary to check drift in the lower extremity unless history and other findings indicate possible lower extremity weakness.[16] When lower extremity evaluation is indicated, the tests should be performed after the prone knee flexion test in Group Fourteen.

Hautant's test is a functional vascular test that employs drift to identify brain stem ischemia due to vertebral artery insufficiency. Since drift is a component of Hautant's test, the procedures are performed simultaneously during testing. Once the initial drift position is achieved, the patient rotates and extends the head to either the right or left. The position is held for 15 to 30 seconds (Fig. 16). The same procedure is repeated for the opposite side. A positive response is pronation and dropping of the hand on the involved side.

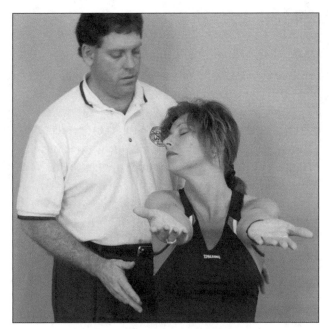

Fig. 16. Combination Testing: Hautant's test and drift test.

If the patient reports no symptoms of vertebral artery ischemia (dizziness, visual disturbances) and pronation with sinking of an extremity does not occur, Hautant's and drift are both negative. If drift does occur, vertebral artery ischemia is suspected. However, other lesions of the cerebrum and brain stem are still possible. In this situation, drift should be tested without head rotation for differential diagnoses.

It is possible for the patient to experience signs of vertebral artery ischemia (dizziness, etc.) without pronation and sinking of either arm. This would be a positive Hautant's test but not a positive drift test.

The finger-to-nose test assesses cerebellar function by determining the accuracy of the patient's movements (coordination). The patient is asked to extend the arms laterally and parallel to the floor. The patient then closes his eyes and alternately touches the nose with the index fingers (Fig. 17: A–C). Movement should be

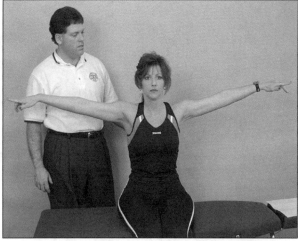

Fig. 17A. Finger-to-nose test starting position.

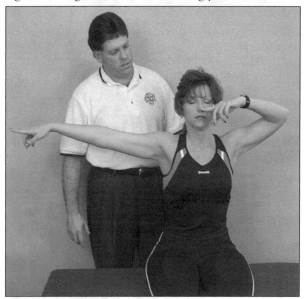

Fig. 17B. Left finger-to-nose test.

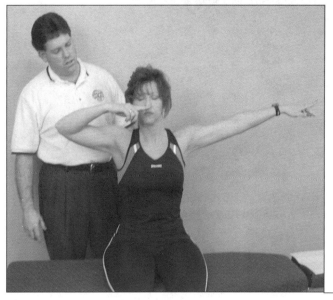

Fig. 17C. Right finger-to-nose test.

31

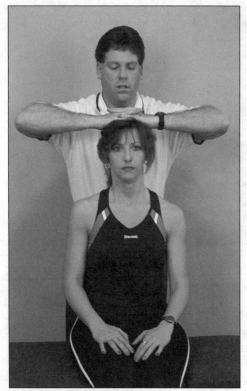

Fig. 18. Cervical Compression Test

quick, smooth and on-target.[3]

Slow cogwheel movements and the inability to accurately touch the nose are positive signs. Coordination testing continues later in the examination with tandem standing in Group Eleven.[1]

The cervical compression test is an effort to reproduce radicular symptoms in the upper extremity, which are due to foramina narrowing in the cervical spine. The examiner applies axial compression to the top of the head with both hands (Fig. 18). Firm pressure is held for approximately five seconds. The test is truly positive only if symptoms are reproduced in the involved extremity. Generalized neck pain is not a positive finding, but it can have clinical significance. Pain from osteoarthritis, facet syndromes or muscle spasm may increase with compression.[17]

The cervical distraction test is an effort to relieve symptoms in the upper extremities that are due to foramina narrowing in the cervical spine. The examiner cups the mastoid processes of the patient's head and applies axial traction for approximately five seconds (Fig. 19). The test is truly positive only if symptoms in the upper extremity are relieved.[17]

Cervical distraction serves as a confirmatory test for cervical compression. Radicular pain produced by cervical compression should be relieved by cervical distraction. Other symptoms caused by cervical compression should also decrease with cervical distraction.

Confirmation of compression and distraction results is also provided by procedures included in Group Nine. These procedures, the brachial plexus tension test and Bakody's test, are supplementary and should be used if compression and distraction are positive or if compression and distraction are negative in the presence of upper extremity complaints. If tests in Groups Four and Nine are all negative in the presence of upper extremity complaints, supplementary procedures for thoracic outlet syndrome in Group Ten should be performed.

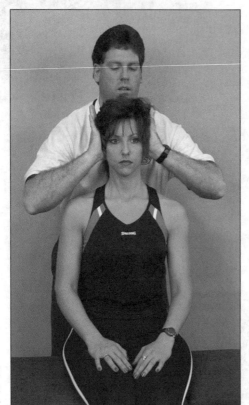

Fig. 19. Cervical Distraction Test

Group Five Tests

1. Hand Grasp
2. Hoffman

Hand grasp is a test for generalized motor strength of the upper extremities. Two testing options are available. Simultaneous hand shaking is the easiest option to perform (Fig. 20A). The second option requires the patient to grasp the examiner's index and middle fingers, and then resist attempts by the examiner to pull away (Fig. 20B). The first test requires the examiner and patient to cross their arms. The second test requires only the examiner's arms to be crossed. Weakness during examination may indicate the need for additional testing of individual muscle groups in the upper extremities.

Hoffman's test is a pathological reflex elicited in the upper extremities and is used for detecting upper motor neuron lesions. This test is equivalent to Babinski's test in the lower extremities. To perform the test, the examiner nips or pinches the nail of the patient's middle finger. Normally, this produces no response. In an individual with an upper motor neuron lesion, flexion occurs at the distal phalanx of the thumb and index finger (Fig. 21: A–C).[18] Babinski and deep tendon reflex testing may help confirm abnormal findings.

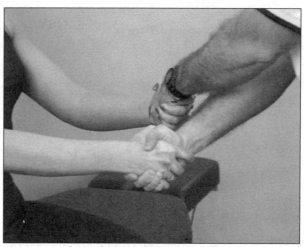

Fig. 20A. Bilateral hand shake for determining grip strength.

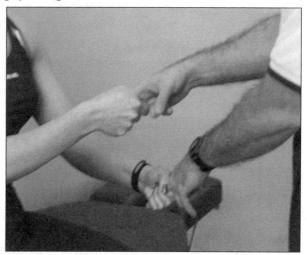

Fig. 20B. Bilateral finger grasp for determining grip strength.

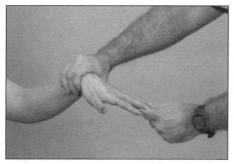

Fig. 21A. Hoffman's Test: starting position.

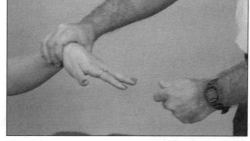

Fig. 21B. Hoffman's Test: normal response.

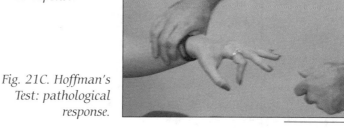

Fig. 21C. Hoffman's Test: pathological response.

Group Six Tests

1. Biceps Reflex
2. Brachioradialis Reflex
3. Triceps Reflex

Deep tendon reflex testing is part of Groups Six and Fourteen. Both groups can be performed with the patient seated. Lower extremity deep tendon reflexes in Group Fourteen will be repeated following the prone knee flexion test in Group Thirteen. The examiner should not record findings until after the tests are repeated.

Deep tendon reflexes are described as normal, hypoactive, hyperactive or absent. Normal reflexes vary between individuals. Some normal patients have little or no reflex response and some have very brisk responses. Symmetry is the key to differentiation in these situations. Symmetry side-to-side and top-to-bottom usually (but not always) indicates reflexes are within normal limits. Symmetrical reflexes should be compared to other findings because symmetry is not a guarantee that pathology is absent.[13]

A hypoactive or absent reflex is indicative of lower motor neuron lesions with absence being the most significant finding. Tapping a tendon more than once, even four to five times, may help identify a diminished reflex. The reflex may be strong with the initial tap, but fatigue with repetition. Hyperactive reflexes are indicative of upper motor neuron lesions. Comparison with other history and exam findings (Hoffman's, Babinski) is always necessary when abnormal reflexes are present.

Biceps, brachioradialis and triceps reflexes test the C5* –C6, C5–C6* and C7 nerve roots. Table 9 details deep tendon reflexes included in Groups Six and Fourteen and their corresponding nerve roots.

Indicates the primary nerve root.

TABLE 9

Deep Tendon Reflexes and Their Corresponding Nerve Roots

Biceps	**C5*-C6**
Brachioradialis	**C5-C6***
Triceps	**C7**
Patellar	**L4**
Achilles	**L5-S1***

Indicates the primary nerve root

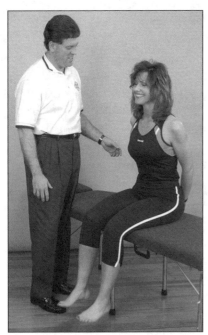

Fig. 22. Slump Test: starting position.

Group Seven Tests

1. Slump
2. Soto-Hall
3. Lindner
4. Lhermette
5. Brudzinski
6. Bechterew
7. SLR
8. CSLR
9. Tripod
10. Kernig
11. Braggard
12. Fajersztajn
13. Valsalva
14. Dejerine

The fourteen tests listed in Group Seven are all accomplished simultaneously by performing the slump test with a few modifications. The slump test is designed to evaluate tension in the neuromeningeal tract from head to toe. Performed in steps, the slump test begins with the seated patient (Fig. 22) flexing the thoracic and lumbar spine, or slumping (Fig. 23). The test proceeds with cervical flexion (Fig. 24), unilateral knee extension (Fig. 25), ankle dorsiflexion (Fig. 26) and cervical exten-

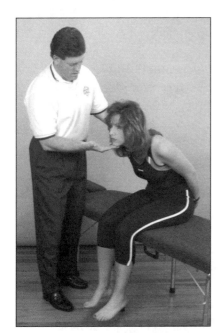

Fig. 23. Slump Test: the slump.

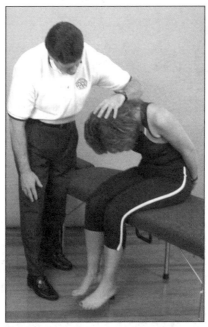

Fig. 24. Slump Test: cervical flexion.

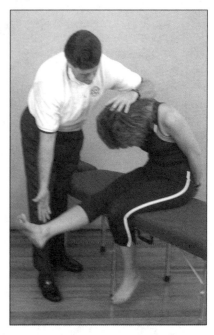

Fig. 25. Slump Test: unilateral knee extension.

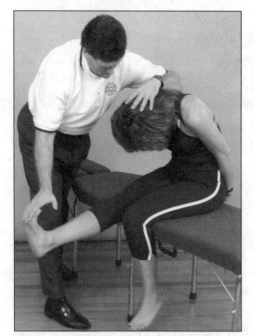

Fig. 26. Slump Test: ankle dorsiflexion.

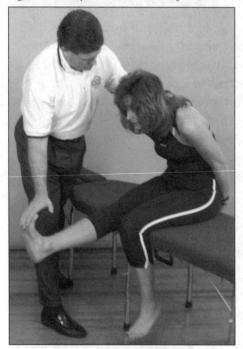

Fig. 27. Slump Test: cervical extension.

*Fig. 28. Slump Test modified
to include bilateral knee extension
and foot dorsiflexion.*

NOTE: This position reproduces the
positions for all of the following tests:
Soto-Hall, Lindner, Lhermette,
Brudzinski, Bechterew, SLR, CSLR,
Kernig, Braggard and Fajersztajn.
Inability to achieve this position
_____ may result in tripod sign.

sion (Fig. 27) in succession. The patient's response is noted with each successive maneuver.[19]

The first four steps gradually increase neuromeningeal tract tension. Cervical extension is performed last to decrease neuromeningeal tension. Reduction of any radicular or spinal cord symptoms produced during the initial steps should be noted.

This test creates discomfort for most asymptomatic individuals due to muscular stretching. This is not a positive finding. True positive findings are neurological, spinal or extremity complaints.

The original slump test reproduces a sitting SLR/Bechterew's test in combination with Braggard's test (foot dorsiflexion) and Lindner's test (cervical flexion). Bechterew's/sitting straight leg raising are both tests for nerve root tension in the involved lower extremity. Braggard's test is another nerve root tension test for the involved lower extremity, usually used to confirm positive Bechterew/SLR results. Braggard's usually intensifies positive findings. The extra stress placed on the nerve by Braggard's can also bring to light positive findings that were sub-sensory or sub-clinical with SLR/Bechterew testing alone.

Lindner's test is for radicular pathologies in the lower extremity. The test is reported to be positive when cervical flexion reproduces radicular signs or sciatica in the lower extremity.

The author modifies the slump test routinely during clinical practice.[20] This increases its efficiency and diagnostic value. Modifications include bilateral knee extension and bilateral foot dorsiflexion (Fig. 28). Dejerine and Valsalva maneuvers can also be added. All of these modifications increase stress on the neuromeningeal tract.

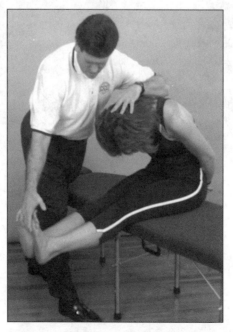

Including both lower extremities adds crossed straight leg raising (CSLR) and Fajersztajn tests to Bechterew/sitting SLR and Braggard. CSLR is also a test for nerve root tension in the lower back and lower extremities. The test is positive if straight leg raising of the uninvolved leg reproduces symptoms in the involved leg. Pain in the symptomatic leg when raising the well leg indicates medial herniation of a disc. Fajersztajn's test is used as a confirmatory test for crossed straight leg raising. Thus, Fajersztajn's is to CSLR what Braggard's is to SLR/Bechterew's. Fajersztajn's can intensify positive findings produced by CSLR or bring to light sub-clinical findings not produced by CSLR testing alone. Beginning with both legs extended is efficient, especially in the absence of radicular complaints in the lower extremities. Positive findings of leg pain must be verified and interpreted by performing extension of the lower extremities unilaterally.

Asking the patient to cough (Dejerine's maneuver) or to bear down as if straining at stool (Valsalva's maneuver) helps rule out or identify space-occupying lesions. Both of these maneuvers increase intrathecal pressure, producing additional stress on the neuromeningeal tract.

Overlapping body mechanics between procedures is of great benefit to the practitioner. In addition to Lindner's test, the cervical flexion component of the slump test reproduces Soto-Hall's test, Lhermette's test and Brudzinski's test. The mechanics are the same for each of these tests. The difference lies in their interpretation. Lindner's is described as positive if lower back or radicular pain is reproduced. Soto-Hall's test is positive for non-specific pain (muscle, ligament or bone pain) in the cervical or thoracic spine. Lhermette's test is for spinal cord pathology and is positive if electric or shock-like sensations course down the upper or lower extremities. Brudzinski's test is positive when cervical flexion causes sharp pain in the back of the neck and/or flexion of the hip and lower extremity. Meningitis, sub-arachnoid hemorrhage or other causes of meningeal irritation can produce a positive Brudzinski's test.

Kernig's test and the tripod sign are also reproduced during the slump test when the patient is flexed by 90 degrees at the waist and the lower extremities are extended. Kernig's test is positive when head, neck or lower back pain prevents the patient from extending the knee, indicating meningeal irritation. Tripod sign is seen when a patient decreases hip flexion in order to extend the knee. The patient typically leans backward, bracing himself on the exam table either to reduce radicular symptoms or due to tight hamstrings. The three legs of the tripod are formed by the patient's buttocks and arms (Fig. 8: A). Differentiation between radicular symptoms and hamstring tightness can be made by determining if symptoms extend below the knee (radicular) and by correlating the result with other neurological findings.

If the patient reports symptoms of meningeal tract irritation, has positive findings for any of the associated tests and/or displays obvious distress during the slump test, the test should be performed again, unmodified, in the steps originally described. If the patient does not experience neurological symptoms or reports only muscular discomfort, the slump test and the related components are all negative (See Table 10).

When the body mechanics of several tests overlap, the tests should be performed once in combination and the results recorded according to the patient's response. No response, or

Practical Examination Strategy:

13. The examination process should take advantage of overlapping body mechanics among procedures. Combining maneuvers increases efficiency.

TABLE 10

Interpretations of component tests reproduced by the slump test or during combination testing, Groups 7 & 16

Patient Position/Mechanics	Response	Positive Test
CERVICAL FLEXION	—Generalized neck and/or thoracic pain/discomfort	Soto-Hall
	—Reproduction of radicular type pain in the symptomatic lower extremity	Lindner's
	—Electric shock sensations unilaterally or bilaterally in the upper and/or lower extremities	Lhermette's
	—Sharp pain in the neck and head and/or flexion of the lower extremities	Brudzinski's
SEATED OR SUPINE WITH HIP FLEXION AND KNEE EXTENSION	—Reproduction of radicular symptoms in the symptomatic lower extremity during testing of the symptomatic lower extemity	Bechterew's/ SLR
	—Reproduction of radicular symptoms in the symptomatic lower extremity during testing of the asymptomatic lower extremity	CSLR
	—Pulling sensation in the posterior thigh and/or inability to fully extend the knees; leaning backwards to extend the knees; no signs/symptoms in the calf or below	Tripod
	—Head, neck or lower back pain prevents knee extension	Kernig's
SEATED OR SUPINE WITH HIP FLEXION, KNEE EXTENSION AND FOOT DORSIFLEXION	—Reproduction or increase of radicular symptoms in the symptomatic lower extremity during testing of the symptomatic lower extemity	Braggard's
	—Reproduction or increase of radicular symptoms in the symptomatic lower extremity during leg testing and foot dorsiflexion of the asymptomatic lower extremity	Fajersztajn
PATIENT APPLIES PRESSURE AGAINST A CLOSED GLOTTIS	—Reproduction of spinal and/or radicular extremity pain	Valsalva
PATIENT COUGHS OR SNEEZES	—Reproduction of spinal and/or radicular extremity pain	Dejerine

an unremarkable response to tests used in combination, usually indicates all tests in that group are negative. Exceptions to this would include repeating or individualizing tests to confirm positive findings or when the patient provides vague or unrealistic responses.

Groups Eight & Twelve Tests

1. Cervical Flexion
2. Cervical Extension
3. Cervical Right Lateral Flexion
4. Cervical Left Lateral Flexion
5. Cervical Right Rotation
6. Cervical Left Rotation
7. Lumbosacral Flexion
8. Lumbosacral Extension
9. Lumbosacral Right Lateral Flexion
10. Lumbosacral Left Lateral Flexion

Range-of-motion testing has changed in several ways over the past decade. Range of motion is no longer the primary factor in determining spinal impairment rating. Inclinometers have replaced goniometers as the standard instrument for range-of-motion measurement. In addition, the numbers listed as normal for the cervical spine region have been revised.[21, 22]

Range of motion is a very subjective or inconsistent objective test. Impairment rating guides list a single set of normal values for each spinal region. No consideration is given to normal variations due to gender or age.[13] It is often difficult to distinguish between limitations due to pain and actual physical limitations. Under certain circumstances, patients move only as far as they choose. Instrumentation provides further inconsistency because many practitioners use devices other than the inclinometers recommended by impairment rating guides. Little or no reliability exists between the dozens of instruments available.[13] Using an instrument for range-of-motion testing is also tedious and time consuming. These characteristics result in a preference for visual estimates by many practitioners.

It is recommended that cervical and lumbosacral ranges of motion be determined by the examiner as other tests and procedures are performed, or that testing be delegated to support staff for completion prior to the doctor's portion of the exam.

During the examination process, several tests provide information regarding spinal range of motion. Hautant's test provides estimates of cervical extension and rotation. The slump test provides an estimation of cervical, thoracic and lumbosacral flexion. Table 11 highlights tests that involve specific spinal ranges of motion.

Once the initial examination is complete, the examiner can record ranges of motion

---

Practical Examination Strategies:

14. An unremarkable or an inappropriate response to tests used in combination usually indicates that all tests in that group are negative.

15. A positive response to any test that has been performed in combination with other tests may indicate a need to perform each test in the group individually.

TABLE 11

SPINAL RANGES OF MOTION AND THEIR RELATIONSHIP TO ORTHOPEDIC AND NEUROLOGICAL TESTS

Movement	Test or Sign
1. Cervical Flexion:	Slump, Soto-Hall, Lindner's, Lhermette's, Brudzinski's, Eden's
2. Cervical Extension:	Hautant, Slump, Adson, Halstead, George's Functional Maneuver, Sphinx
3. Cervical Lateral Flexion:	Brachial Plexus Tension Test, Shoulder Distraction
4. Cervical Rotation:	Hautant, Adson, Halstead, George's Functional Maneuver
5. Lumbosacral Flexion:	Slump, Bechterew's, SLR, CSLR, Kernig, Knee Bends
6. Lumbosacral Extension:	Sphinx, Nachlas
7. Lumbar Lateral Flexion:	Kemp's

based on observations made during the exam. If visual estimates are used, it is best that the patient be re-evaluated by the same examiner. This provides a degree of consistency between exams. If a different practitioner will be evaluating the patient, it is better to use instrumentation.[13] Instrumentation can be performed by support staff who also record weight, height, blood pressure and temperature prior to the doctor's portion of the exam. Space is provided on the sample exam form from Appendix B to record measured or observed findings.

In addition to the actual degrees for each range of motion, three other factors should be identified and recorded: aberrant motion, crepitus and pain. Aberrant motion refers to the manner or rhythm in which the patient moves through a plane of motion. Movement through a plane of motion should be smooth if normal. Cogwheel or ratchet- like motions can indicate muscle or joint dysfunction. Deviation into another axis of movement may also indicate muscle or joint dysfunction.

Although our assessment does not include the tempromandibular joint, active movements of the TMJ provide a good example of aberrant movement during range of motion. During normal opening and closing of the mouth, the mentum (center of the chin) should remain in line with the mid–sagittal plane of the head. The nose can be used as a reference point. If the mentum deviates to one side and back (C-type curve) upon opening, hypomobility is present in the joint on the side of the deviation.[1] If deviation occurs back and forth (S-type curve), then musculature imbalance or condylar displacement are present.[1] Muscle spasm, disc problems and capsulitis can also cause aberrant motion of the TMJ.[1]

Abnormal rhythm during range of motion can occur in several regions and joints of the body. McGee[1] refers to these movements as "trick" movements. McNabb[2] describes reversal of lumbopelvic rhythm during examination of the lower back. Patients with disc degeneration and posterior joint lesions typically bend the knees and tuck the pelvis underneath the spine in order to move from a flexed to a standing position. Serial drawings of this phenomenon actually appear on the cover of McNabb's text.

The tripod test described under Group Seven provides an example of aberrant motion. The seated patient with nerve root tension in a lower extremity or with tight ham-strings will lean backwards in order to achieve full extension of the extremity. The patient forms a tripod with the buttocks and arms, this sign is also referred to as the "flip" sign. The author has noted that, during examination of the cervical spine, the head will move to one side and back or side to side when the patient moves from full flexion to full extension. This can be a result of strain, sprain, muscle imbalance or subluxation.

Common sense would dictate that abnormal rhythm during range of motion would most likely be present in combination with reduced range of motion. However, it is possible to have abnormal rhythm with full range of motion. In these situations, how the patient achieves full range of motion is more important than whether or not he achieves full range of motion.

Any cracking or creaking sound or sensation noted during the movement of a joint, muscle or tendon is termed crepitus.[23] Chiropractors and their patients are familiar with the crepitus associated with various types of manipulation. Bubbles of nitrogen gas within synovial joints pop when the joint shifts or is manipulated. This type of crepitus can also be noted by the patient during routine movements in daily activities. Once the bubble "pops," it takes time for the gas to coalesce, reforming the bubble. Thus, crepitus that cannot immediately be reproduced is usually from a synovial joint. Crepitus that is repeatable is usually due to tight muscles/tendons repeatedly snapping over a joint. Crepitus from tight muscles/tendons is often benign, but can become pathological due to friction. Friction leads to tendonitis or bursitis. Repeated crepitus can also be due to joint derangement or a loose fragment within the joint. Derangement of a knee menis-cus produces the repetitive crepitus noted with McMurray's test.[1]

Patients often provide descriptions of crepitus during the history-taking process. They describe crepitus as popping, grinding, cracking or rubbing sounds. Patients can feel and hear crepitus. Examiners can often palpate crepitus, and in some cases the examiner can hear crepitus. In any case, the examiner should always record the patient's reports of crepitus even if it is not identifiable by objective means.

Space has been provided on the exam form to record findings of crepitus during spinal ranges of motion in Groups Eight and Twelve. Space has also been provided under deep knee bend testing in Group Eleven. Findings of repeated crepitus in Group Eleven should be correlated with muscle tension findings for the lower extremities recorded under observations in Group Three.

Pain during active range of motion traditionally indicates musculature involvement. Pain during passive range of motion traditionally indicates ligamentous involvement. Combinations of the two are possible and frequent. Pain during active range of motion will be recorded with range of motion. Pain during passive range of motion will be recorded with palpation.

Group Nine Tests

1. Brachial Plexus Tension
2. Bakody

The brachial plexus tension test and Bakody's test are supplementary procedures performed to confirm positive results of cervical compression and distraction tests. They are also performed when cervical compression and distraction are negative in the presence of upper extremity complaints. There is no need for the brachial plexus or Bakody's test if upper extremity complaints are not reported and compression and distraction are negative.

Very few orthopedic or neurological tests are pathognomonic. This makes it necessary to perform more than one test for most suspected pathologies. Two or more tests for most common spinal pathologies are included in the Practical Examination. Some tests are actually repeated with the patient in different positions to verify results. Confirming results, whether positive or negative, is a very important aspect of orthopedic and neurological evaluations.

Brachial plexus tension and Bakody's tests are similar to cervical compression and distraction tests in that the first step of each pair attempts to reproduce radicular pain and the second attempts to relieve it.

The brachial plexus tension test places the brachial plexus and the cervical nerve roots in traction. To perform the test, the examiner abducts the patient's arm slightly behind the coronal plane. The glenohumeral joint is then externally rotated, the elbow is extended and the forearm is supinated. Extension of the wrist with lateral and forward flexion of the cervical spine to the opposite side of testing can be added to increase tension on the plexus and nerve roots. If radicular complaints are reproduced, flexion of the elbow should relieve the symptoms[1] (Fig. 29: A–C).

Bakody's test is performed by asking the patient to place the palm of his hand on the top of his head (Fig. 30). The patient with radicular complaints often reports a reduction of symptoms. This test is remarkable when positive. Patients may describe a positive Bakody's sign during the history process by reporting that the only relief they can obtain is by elevating their arm above their head. Elevating the arm above the head is

Practical Examination Strategy:

16. Tests that confirm or reinforce the results of other tests should be included in the examination process.

often described as the only comfortable position in which the patient can sleep. Simultaneously testing the left and right sides increases testing efficiency (Fig. 31).

Patients with thoracic outlet syndrome due to neurovascular compression by the pectoralis minor muscle (hyperabduction syndrome) may report exacerbation of symptoms with Bakody's maneuver. Sleeping with the arm elevated for these patients often exacerbates symptoms (a positive Wright's sign).

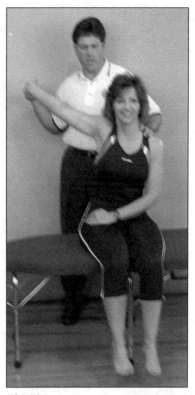

Fig 29A.
Brachial Plexus Tension Test

Group Ten Tests

1. Adson's
2. Halstead's
3. Wright's
4. Eden's
5. George's Functional Maneuver

Group Ten consists of four tests for thoracic outlet syndrome and one test for vertebral artery compromise. The tests are supplementary (used only to confirm or rule out other exam findings). There is no need for the thoracic outlet syndrome tests in the absence of upper extremity complaints or if tests for nerve root tension reproduce the patient's symptoms. If tests for radicular pathology are negative in the presence of upper extremity complaints, then thoracic outlet syndrome testing should be performed.

George's Functional Maneuver is used to confirm a positive Hautant's test from Group Four. In the absence of a positive Hautant's test or other cardiovascular risk factors, the test is not performed.

Adson's, Halstead's and George's Functional Maneu-

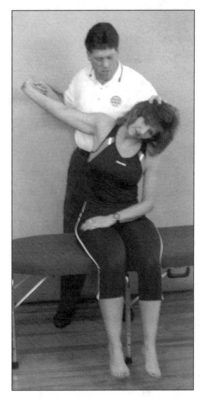

Fig. 29B.
Cervical, lateral and forward flexion with wrist extension.

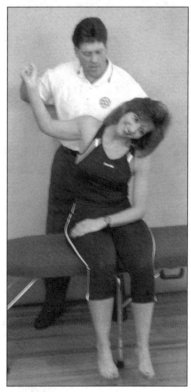

Fig. 29C.
Elbow flexion to reduce radicular pain.

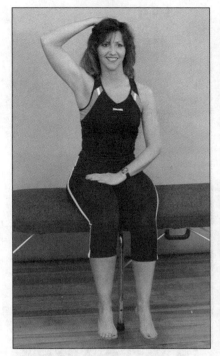

Fig. 30. Bakody's Test

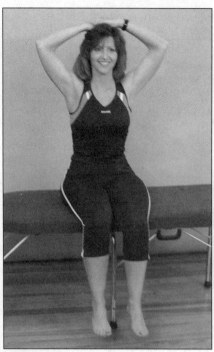

Fig. 31. Bilateral Bakody's Test

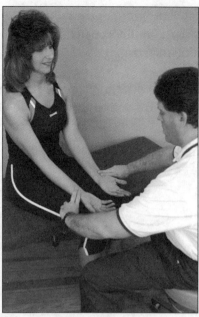

Fig. 32. Bilateral palpation of the radial pulses: starting position for Adson's, Halstead's, George's Functional Maneuver and Eden's Tests.

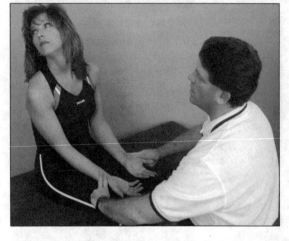

Fig. 33. Right Adson's test, left Halstead's test and right George's Functional Maneuver.

ver can be performed simultaneously. The examiner should sit or stand directly in front of the patient and palpate the radial pulse bilaterally (Fig. 32). The patient is instructed to rotate and extend the head and neck to the right. This is a right Adson's test, a left Halstead's test and a right George's Functional Maneuver (Fig. 33). After holding this position for 10 to 20 seconds, the procedure is repeated with head and neck rotation and extension to the opposite side.

Adson's test screens for compression of the neurovascular bundle by the scalene muscles and/or a cervical rib. A change in pulse amplitude and frequency on the side of head/neck rotation is a positive finding. Reproduction of the patient's upper extremity signs and symptoms is also a positive finding.

Halstead's test screens for traction of the neurovascular bundle by the scalene muscles on the side opposite of head/neck rotation. Reproduction of the patient's upper extremity signs and symptoms or a decrease in pulse amplitude and frequency are positive findings.

George's Functional Maneuver employs rotation and extension of the head and neck to produce stress on the vertebral arteries. The test position reduces blood flow in both vertebral arteries, with the greatest reduction and flow occurring in the artery on the opposite side of rotation.[24] Dizziness and nystagmus are positive findings.

Progressing from Adson's, Halstead's and George's tests to Eden's test is easy, because Eden's test also requires bilateral palpation of the radial pulse. Starting positions for the patient and examiner remain the same (Fig. 32).

For Eden's test the patient is instructed to pull the shoulders posterior and inferior, protruding the chest (Fig. 34A). This position is similar to standing at attention, thus the reference to "soldier's test."[11] The patient is then instructed to flex the chin to the chest (Fig. 34B). Decreased amplitude or frequency of the radial pulse indicates compression of the neurovascular bundle between the first rib and clavicle.

Wright's test requires a shift in examiner position from in front of to behind the patient. The examiner begins by unilaterally palpating the radial pulse. With the arm fully extended and held slightly posterior, the examiner abducts the extremity to at least 120 degrees (Fig. 35). A decrease in pulse amplitude is a positive sign indicating compression of the neurovascular bundle under the insertion of the pectoralis minor muscle. The procedure is then performed on the opposite side. While recording the results of any examination that includes Adson's, Halstead's, Eden's or Wright's test, be sure to include findings for the radial pulse in Group Seventeen.

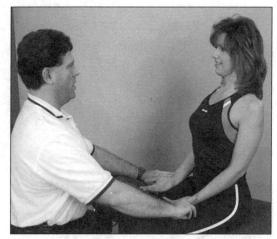
Fig. 34A. Eden's Test: starting position.

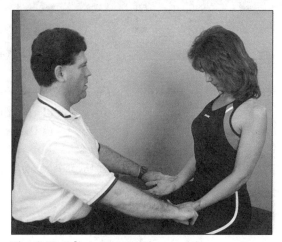
Fig. 34B. Eden's Test: testing position.

Group Eleven Tests

1. Knee Bends
2. Toe Raises
3. Heel Standing
4. Tandem Stance

With the exception of height and weight measurement in Group One, the procedures in Groups Eleven and Twelve are the only procedures that require the patient to stand. Standing procedures may require close supervision by the examiner because painful lumbopelvic and lower extremity conditions may render the patient unstable. Balance and coordination problems due to age or central nervous system pathology may also cause instability. In addition to examiner assistance, a handrail or sturdy examination table can be used by the patient for stabilization if necessary.

Deep knee bends provide quick assessment of lower

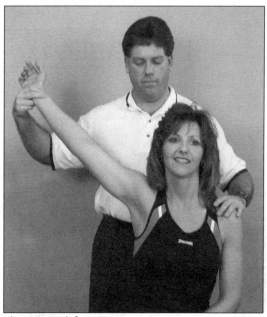
Fig. 35. Wright's Test

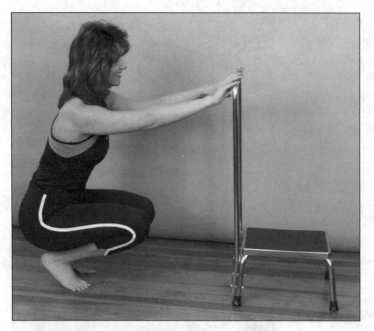

*Fig. 36. Deep
Knee Bend*

extremity range of motion and motor function related to the L2 through S2 nerve roots. Flexion and extension of the hip, knee and ankle joints are required for deep knee bends. The exam is rapid and provides bilateral comparison (Fig. 36). Magee[1] describes a similar procedure as the "quick test."[1] Deep knee bends should be performed five or more times to assist the examiner in determining lower extremity ROM, differentiating causes of lower extremity crepitus and identifying muscle weakness.

If the patient can perform deep knee bends, there is little or no reason to assess ROM for each lower extremity joint. Crepitus from synovial joints usually occurs once at the onset of motion and does not occur again until nitrogen gas bubbles and synovial fluid have time to coalesce again. Repetitive crepitus during joint motion is usually due to tight muscles and tendons. An exception would be crepitus in the knee joint due to meniscus pathology. Weakness of a muscle or group of muscles may not become evident with a single contraction. Performing five or more repetitions is necessary to help rule out weakness.

Table 12 provides a description of lower extremity movements and their corresponding innervations. Note that each movement requires the effort of two successive nerve roots, and that the two opposite motions at each joint require four consecutive nerve roots.[25] This pattern provides for easy memorization of root levels and their corresponding actions.

TABLE 12

Motor innervation for lower extremity movements performed during deep knee bends	
Movement	**Nerve Root Level**
HIP	
flexion	L2-L3
extension	L4-L5
KNEE	
extension	L3-L4
flexion	L5-S1
ANKLE	
dorsiflexion	L4-L5
planar flexion	S1-S2

Heel walking and toe walking are standard motor tests for assessing the L4–L5 and S1–S2 nerve roots, respectively. Toe raises are recommended over toe walking because the test localizes the muscles tested and allows better stabilization of the patient. The patient can hold on to a stationary object, or the examiner can "spot" the patient during toe raising (Fig. 37: A–B). McNab[2] recommends unilateral toe raises with 10 repetitions. Unilateral performance provides further isolation, and the repetitions are to assist in identifying weakness. Twenty-five bilateral toe raises are recommended in this exam for patient safety and stability. The extra 15 toe raises are to fatigue compensation provided by the normal side when unilateral weakness is present.

Standing in place on the heels for 15 seconds is recommended as a substitute for heel walking, again for stabilization purposes (Fig. 38). Heel standing is maintained for a full 15 seconds in order to induce fatigue in weak anterior leg muscles innovated by the L4–L5 nerve roots.

Patients without muscle weakness can easily perform knee bends, toe raises and heel standing. Weakness, cramps and/or fasciculations are positive signs of pathology for any of the three tests.

Walking in tandem (heel-to-toe in a straight line) is a standard test of coordination. The inability to walk in tandem may be an indication of an intracranial lesion. Standing in tandem is recommended as a substi-

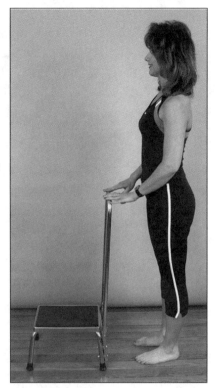

Fig. 37A. Starting position for toe raises.

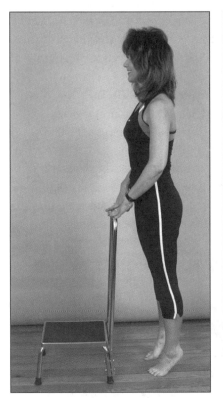

Fig. 37B. Toe raises.

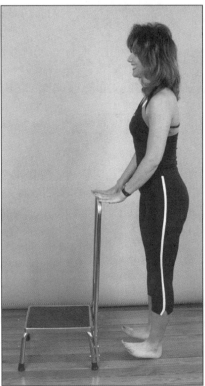

Fig. 38. Standing on the heels.

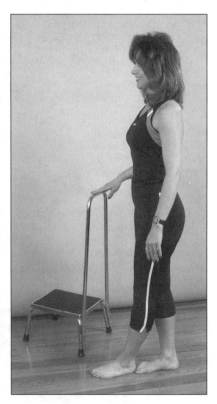

Fig. 39. Tandem stance

tute for walking in tandem, because standing in tandem is more difficult to perform (Fig. 39).[1] It is also easier for the examiner to stabilize the patient should he begin to fall. Standing in tandem is the second check for coordination in the examination process. Finger-to-nose testing for the upper extremity was included in Group Four.

Group Thirteen Tests

1. Hibbs
2. Sphinx
3. Nachlas
4. Femoral Stretch
5. Prone Knee Flexion

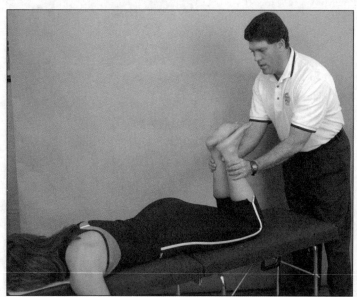

Fig. 40A. Hibbs Test: starting position.

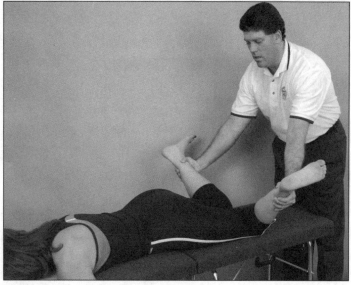

Fig. 40B. Bilateral Hibbs Test

Patient positioning is switched now from standing to lying prone. The first five prone procedures can be performed in two steps. Hibbs test is performed individually while the remaining tests in Group Thirteen (Sphinx, Nachlas, femoral stretch and prone knee flexion) are performed simultaneously. Hibbs test is performed with the patient lying prone. The examiner grasps the lower legs near the foot/ankle and passively flexes the patient's knees to 90 degrees (Fig. 40A). Once this position is achieved the examiner uses the lower leg as a lever to internally rotate the femurs (Fig. 40B). Pain and/or decreased internal rotation are positive findings for hip joint pathology.

Isolation of the hip joint is easy to achieve with Hibbs test, and the test can be performed for the left and right sides at the same time. Both of these facts make Hibbs test a better choice than Patrick's test for hip joint pathology. In addition, Hibbs test evaluates the hip for decreased or restricted internal rotation, which is thought to be one of the earliest signs of hip joint pathology.[26] Patrick's test evaluates external rotation of the hip. Patrick's test also stresses the ipsilateral SI joint during testing, making it harder to interpret reports of pain.[27] Patrick's test should be used as a confirmatory test to Hibbs.

The four remaining tests in Group Thirteen will be performed simultaneously by combining the Sphinx position and the position required for prone knee flexion. This position will then be held for approximately one minute.

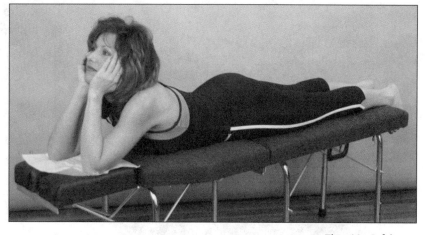

Fig. 41. Sphinx Test

The Sphinx test is a prone measurement of lumbosacral extension (normal equals 25 degrees). The test is performed by having the prone patient prop himself up on his elbows and rest his chin in his hands (Fig. 41). This position is usually held for at least 20 seconds.[1] It is recommended that the position be held for approximately one minute in order to complete the prone knee flexion test simultaneously. It is worth noting that the Sphinx position also creates extension of the cervical spine and can cause facet joint irritation at multiple levels. Mild stenosis may be induced in the cervical and lumbar regions with the Sphinx position due to buckling of ligamentous structures. Stenosis will be important in the prone knee flexion test.

Prone knee flexion is a test for identifying occult disc protrusion causing spinal nerve irritation. The conditions are occult in that the patient's reports of leg pain are accompanied by minimal or no motor weakness or reflex asymmetry. Other objective findings, such as straight leg raising, may also be negative. Prone knee flexion seeks to enhance or produce objective findings by extending the lumbar spine, exaggerating stenosis. The test is accomplished by hyperflexing the patient's knees so the heels approximate the buttocks while lying prone (Fig. 42). This position is held for one minute. After 60 seconds, flexion of the knees is reduced and patellar and Achilles reflexes are performed (Fig. 43).

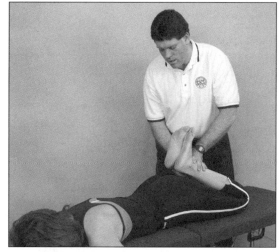

Fig. 42. Prone Knee Flexion Test

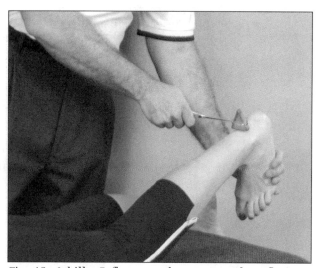

Fig. 43. Achilles Reflex: secondary to prone knee flexion.

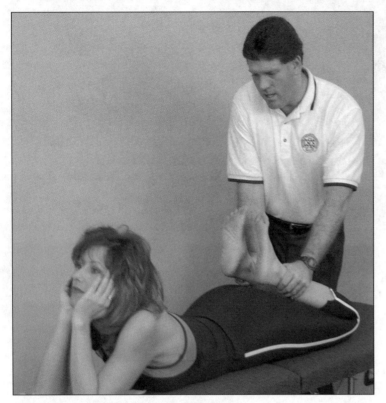

Motor testing of the extensor hallucis longus, tibialis anterior and gastrocnemius/soleus muscles can also be utilized following reflex testing. Positive findings are reflex asymmetry or motor weakness.[28]

Flexion of a patient's knees while in a prone posture is the same mechanism required for the Nachlas and femoral stretch tests.

Nachlas test is positive if knee hyperflexion produces pain in the SI joints or the lumbosacral junction. The femoral stretch test is positive if knee hyperflexion produces pain or paresthesia in the anterior thigh along the distribution of the femoral nerve.

Combining the Sphinx and prone knee flexion positions (Fig. 44) can produce a

Fig. 44. Combination Testing: Sphinx and prone knee flexion tests.

variety of patient responses. The ability to interpret these responses and determine positive vs. negative results for several tests (as with the slump test) separates the doctors from the technicians. Table 8 lists patient responses to the combined maneuvers and their meanings.

TABLE 8

Interpretation of Patient Responses to Group Thirteen	
Location of Symptom	**Meaning**
Pain in the cervical region	Cervical facet syndrome
Lower back pain	Positive Sphinx
Pain at the lumbosacral junction	Positive Nachlas
Pain in either SI joint	Positive Nachlas
Pulling/stretching sensation in the anterior thigh	Tight quadriceps muscles
Pain or paresthesia in the anterior thigh along the course of the femoral nerve	Positive femoral stretch test
Post-testing loss or decrease in reflex and/or motor function in the home leg	Positive prone knee flexion test

Group Fourteen Tests

1. Achilles
2. Patellar
3. Babinski

Interpretation of deep tendon reflexes has already been described under Group Six. Emphasis here is on repeating the Achilles and patellar reflexes after the prone knee flexion test to detect occult nerve irritation due to disc protrusion. A difference in pre- and post-results (reduced or lost reflexes) is a positive prone knee flexion test.

Patellar and Achilles reflexes test the L4 and L5-S1 nerve roots. Table 9 details deep tendon reflexes, including those in Groups Fourteen and Six and their corresponding nerve roots.

Babinski's test is the most common test for upper motor neuron lesions. The test is easy to perform with the Achilles and patellar reflexes following prone knee flexion. Babinski's test is performed by stroking the plantar aspect of the foot with the pointed handle of the reflex hammer (Fig. 45). A positive response is flaring and extension of the toes (Fig. 46). Results should be correlated with Hoffman's sign and deep tendon reflex testing.

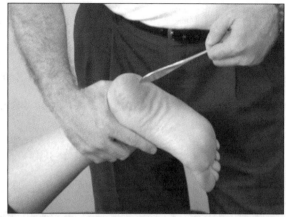

Fig. 45. Babinski's Test

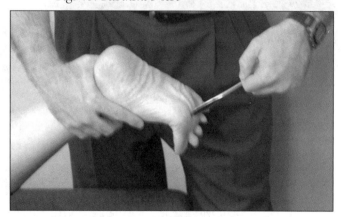

Fig. 46. Pathological Babinski's Response

TABLE 9

Deep Tendon Reflexes and Their Corresponding Nerve Roots	
Biceps	C5*-C6
Brachioradialis	C5-C6*
Triceps	C7
Patellar	L4
Achilles	L5-S1*

*Indicates the primary nerve root

Group Fifteen Tests

1. Palpation of Spinal and Pelvic Joints
2. Palpation of Spinal Musculature
3. Fluid Motion Test

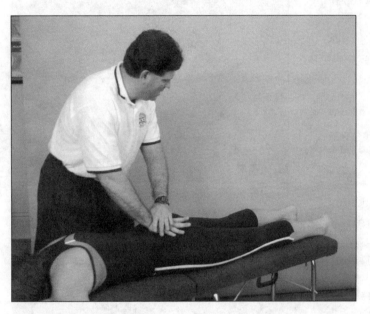

Fig. 47. Fluid Motion Test

Muscle tone, spasm, trigger points, swelling, joint play, crepitus and joint end feel are among the many musculoskeletal findings that can be identified by palpation. While each of these factors is important, this exam will only utilize palpation for screening certain joint and muscle dysfunctions in the spinal and pelvic regions. Dysfunction may involve hypermobility or hypomobility (fixation). Dysfunction and pain for each spinal region (cervical, thoracic, lumbar) is recorded as occurring in the upper, middle or lower aspect of each region. Distinction can also be made between left, right or bilateral findings. Pelvic joint dysfunction can be recorded at the lumbosacral junction, the left SI joint, the right SI joint or the coccyx.

The fluid motion test is an excellent test for determining sacroiliac joint dysfunction. The test is performed by applying firm, steady pressure through the plane of the sacroiliac joint or the sacroiliac articulation of a prone patient (Fig. 47). The test is negative if only the leg on the side being tested elongates. The test is positive if both legs extend the same amount. A positive test indicates joint fixation (hypomobility) of the side being tested. The test is then repeated on the opposite side.[29]

The author prefers the fluid motion test over the knee-raiser test, as fluid motion tests passive range of motion (joint play) over active range of motion. Fluid motion also offers a more secure testing position (prone) than knee-raiser (standing) for patients in acute distress. Fluid motion also provides a direct evaluation of SI joint dysfunction compared to the indirect information obtained from leg length analysis. Fluid motion testing is also less affected by factors that may interfere with leg length analysis, such as amputation, congenital leg length deficiencies or trauma/disease-induced leg length deficiencies.

Abnormal muscle tonicity can be described as hypotonic, hypertonic, spasmodic and/or painful for each spinal level. Again, distinction within each region, and right, left or bilateral findings, can be identified.

Group Sixteen Tests

1. Soto-Hall
2. Lindner
3. Lhermette
4. Brudzinski
5. SLR
6. CSLR
7. Kernig
8. Braggard
9. Fajersztajn
10. Valsalva
11. Dejerine

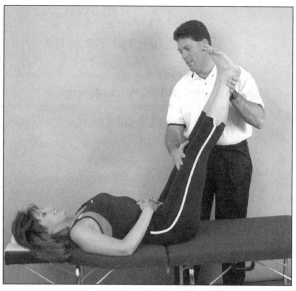

Fig. 48. Combination Testing: bilateral SLR, CSLR and Kernig's tests.

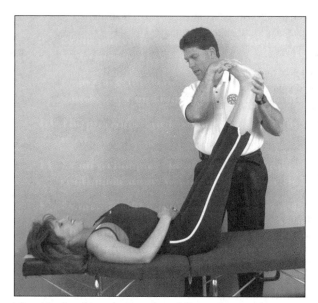

Fig. 49. Combination Testing: bilateral SLR, CSLR, Kernig's, Braggard's and Fajersztajn's tests.

The final two series of tests, Groups Sixteen and Seventeen, consist of supplementary procedures. They are also the only procedures in the examination routine that are performed with the patient in the supine position. Tests in Group Sixteen have already been discussed in Group Seven. The interpretation of these procedures remains the same. Only the patient positioning has changed. It is not necessary to perform the tests in Group Sixteen if they are negative in Group Seven and lower extremity complaints are not present. Group Sixteen procedures can be performed if procedures in Group Seven are positive; this will help confirm results. If the tests in Group Seven were negative in the presence of lower extremity symptoms, Group Sixteen should be performed to confirm negative findings and to help rule out malingering.

The eleven tests included in Group Sixteen are performed simultaneously. The examiner performs bilateral straight leg raising to approximately 70 degrees (SLR, CSLR, Kernig) (Fig. 48). The examiner then dorsiflexes both feet (Braggard, Fajersztajn) (Fig. 49). The patient is now instructed to flex his chin and neck toward his chest (Soto-Hall, Lindner, Lhermette, Brudzinski) (Fig. 50) and bear down (Valsalva). After the Valsalva maneuver is released, the same position is repeated with the patient coughing (Dejerine). Positive findings for the combination of tests in Group Sixteen require reproduction of the patient's chief complaints and assigning the patient's response to the appropriate test (Table 10).

Practical Examination Strategies:

17. Testing procedures, which can be performed utilizing more than one patient position, should be performed first in the position most likely to produce positive results.

18. The examination process should include methods for identifying malingering and non-organic conditions.

TABLE 10

Interpretations of component tests reproduced by the slump test or during combination testing, Groups 7 & 16

Patient Position/Mechanics	Response	Positive Test
CERVICAL FLEXION	—Generalized neck and/or thoracic pain/discomfort	Soto-Hall
	—Reproduction of radicular type pain in the symptomatic lower extremity	Lindner's
	—Electric shock sensations unilaterally or bilaterally in the upper and/or lower extremities	Lhermette's
	—Sharp pain in the neck and head and/or flexion of the lower extremities	Brudzinski's
SEATED OR SUPINE WITH HIP FLEXION AND KNEE EXTENSION	—Reproduction of radicular symptoms in the symptomatic lower extremity during testing of the symptomatic lower extemity	Bechterew's/ SLR
	—Reproduction of radicular symptoms in the symptomatic lower extremity during testing of the asymptomatic lower extremity	CSLR
	—Pulling sensation in the posterior thigh and/or inability to fully extend the knees; leaning backwards to extend the knees; no signs/symptoms in the calf or below	Tripod
	—Head, neck or lower back pain prevents knee extension	Kernig's
SEATED OR SUPINE WITH HIP FLEXION, KNEE EXTENSION AND FOOT DORSIFLEXION	—Reproduction or increase of radicular symptoms in the symptomatic lower extremity during testing of the symptomatic lower extemity	Braggard's
	—Reproduction or increase of radicular symptoms in the symptomatic lower extremity during leg testing and foot dorsiflexion of the asymptomatic lower extremity	Fajersztajn
PATIENT APPLIES PRESSURE AGAINST A CLOSED GLOTTIS	—Reproduction of spinal and/or radicular extremity pain	Valsalva
PATIENT COUGHS OR SNEEZES	—Reproduction of spinal and/or radicular extremity pain	Dejerine

Tests may be individualized if necessary to confirm results. Reports of general discomfort, as with the slump test, are not positive findings.

A clinical test should be performed in the position most likely to elicit a positive result. Repeating the test in a secondary position may provide confirmation of the previous finding and/or information regarding the severity of injury. This is the reason for performing the modified slump test prior to or instead of supine procedures for disc and nerve root pathology in Group Sixteen.

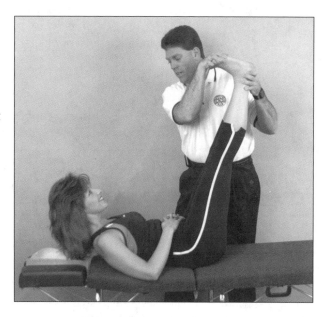

Kemp's test for disc and radicular pathology can be performed with the patient standing or seated. Since there is more pressure in the lumbar intervertebral discs when seated,[30] disc pathology is more likely to be identified with the patient in this position. Straight leg raising should be more diagnostic for disc pathology when performed sitting versus lying supine for this same reason. Another example of this principle is seen in testing the medial and collateral ligaments of the knee. These ligaments can be tested with the knee in a variety of positions between 30 degrees of flexion and complete extension. Instability of these ligamentous structures is more likely to be detected with the knee partially flexed, as opposed to fully extended. Testing should begin in the partially flexed position.

Fig. 50. Combination Testing: bilateral SLR, CSLR, Kernig's, Braggard's, Fajersztajn's, Soto-Hall's, Lindner's, Lhermette's and Brudzinski's tests.

True malingering is not very common, and when it does occur, suspicions are often confirmed during the routine history and examination process. Several tests (SLR, CSLR, Soto-Hall, etc.) can be repeated in the rapid assessment examination to help confirm initial results and possibly identify unrealistic responses. Patients with a positive SLR in the seated position should have a similar response while lying supine. If the responses are very different, the examiner should be alert to the possibility of non-organic conditions. There are a variety of orthopedic and neurological tests meant to identify or rule out such conditions. These tests are best used as supplementary procedures and do not have to be part of every examination.

Group Seventeen Tests

1. Radial Pulse
2. Posterior Tibial Pulse

When upper or lower extremity complaints are reported, yet tests for disc and radicular pathology are negative, pulses should be evaluated. This is especially true for older patients because cardiovascular conditions may be responsible for extremity symptoms.

Coronary artery disease can produce upper extremity complaints. Thoracic outlet syndromes can cause upper extremity symptoms (See Group Thirteen). Aortic aneurysms can cause upper and lower extremity symptoms. Leg pain can result from Buerger's disease and intermittent or neurogenic clandication.

Palpation of the radial and posterior tibial pulses will not specifically identify any of these conditions, but is a good starting place. Further evaluation by measuring blood pressure in the extremity (upper or lower) and Doppler studies may be advised.

When upper extremity symptoms are present and tests for radicular pathology are negative, tests for thoracic outlet syndrome are performed. Tests for thoracic outlet syndrome involve palpation of the radial pulse. Since the procedure has already been performed, the only extra step required is recording the results.

If lower extremity symptoms are present and tests for radicular pathology are negative, palpation of the posterior tibial pulse is performed. Bilateral comparison to determine if pulses are strong, weak or absent is quick and easy (Fig. 51). While a weak or absent pulse is considered a sign of possible pathology, a strong pulse does not guarantee the absence of pathology. Further evaluation may still be necessary.

The ability to perform the posterior tibial pulse test is another reason for the patient to have bare feet. Palpation of the dorsalis pedis pulse was not selected for the exam, as this artery is often congenitally absent.[31]

Nine Minutes, 55 Seconds

The description of the *Practical Assessment of the Chiropractic Patient* is complete. The basic exam without supplementary procedures covers 70 orthopedic and neurological tests in 10 minutes or less. With supplementary procedures, up to 90 tests are performed. Initial attempts to perform the examination as described will require more than 10 minutes. With practice, the process will fit within the recommended 10-minute time frame, even with supplementary procedures.

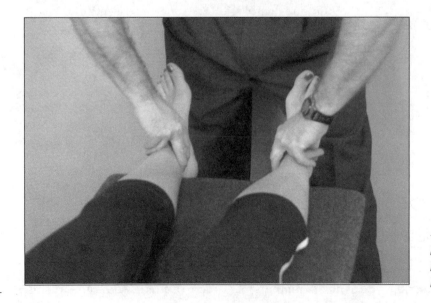

Fig. 51. Bilateral palpation of the posterior tibial pulses.

ADDITIONAL TESTS

Radiographs, advanced imaging and laboratory tests typically follow the physical examination. Care should be taken to assure the need for additional tests is borne by the exam. Some practitioners have developed a habit of ordering MR scans and other advanced diagnostics for every workers'-compensation or personal-injury patient, regardless of the history and physical findings. In today's environment of "managed cost" and prolific precertification, this practice is being challenged. Documenting the necessity of any test, especially if it is expensive or invasive, is now paramount.

PROGRESS EVALUATIONS

In any process, feedback to determine if outcomes are progressing as expected is important. This is true of chiropractic care because the majority of the time, treatment is a process – not a single event. Progress evaluations subsequent to initial evaluation will consist of rechecking previous positive findings and other procedures (bullets) required to justify the level of CPT codes utilized (See Tables 5 and 6).

Coding for the routine progress exam will likely fall one code level below the initial level of service since fewer procedures are required; for example, a 99204 initial exam followed by a 99213 progress exam. If the patient fails to respond, experiences a new complaint or injury or has an exacerbation, it is recommended that the entire initial evaluation and any other necessary tests be performed. In these situations the progress exam code level should be consistent with the initial level; for example, a 99204 initial exam followed by a 99214 progress exam. Always cross-reference progress exam content to CPT coding requirements.

Positive findings from the initial evaluation form can be summarized on a separate form or travel card to be rechecked at a later date. This will avoid the necessity of having to pull the patient's entire file to find the initial exam form. Assuming the patient is progressing as expected, there is usually no need to recheck tests that were previously negative. Doctors performing utilization reviews often see progress evaluations that involve rechecking every test. In some cases the second or third exam will document a positive finding that was initially negative. This gives the appearance that chiropractic care is creating new pathologies. Consider the following: If a patient presents for medical evaluation of digestive complaints, he may be subjected to a multitude of diagnostic tests. Stomach, liver, gall bladder and intestinal function may be examined. Once the condition is localized to the gall bladder, for example, it is unlikely that progress evaluations will include anything other than functional tests for the gall bladder. It would not be necessary, efficient or cost-effective to recheck the other organs.

Practical Examination Strategy:

19. Physical examination procedures should establish the reasoning behind ordering or not ordering additional tests, such as imaging or lab studies.

Practical
Examination
Strategy:

20.Exam
procedures
should be
applicable for
both new and
established
patient
evaluations.

New-patient and progress examinations are usually scheduled. However, spontaneous situations often occur. New patients may request emergency service and established patients may experience sudden changes in symptoms or new chief complaints. Inevitably these situations occur when the doctor is very busy. The evaluation described above provides an efficient exam process that can be performed in a time frame that will not completely disrupt the entire schedule.

Portions of the exam process can also be used to double-check patients who have the same complaints as before and are requesting a maintenance or check-up adjustment.

A good update for a routine or maintenance patient might include the tests in Group One (constitutional signs), Group Four (Hautant's, drift, cervical compression, cervical distraction, etc.) and Group Seven (slump test). This update would provide a great deal of information in a short amount of time.

Periodic progress evaluations are vital for several reasons. The doctor needs feedback to determine if care is progressing as expected or should be altered or discontinued. The patient knows how he feels, but is often more interested in how the doctor views his progress. The patient needs reassurance that he is improving. If improvement is not seen, the patient needs reassurance that the doctor has an alternate plan.

Re-evaluation of the patient's progress also provides documentation for insurance carriers, employers, other health care providers, caseworkers, utilization reviewers, attorneys, judges and many others who have an interest in the patient's progress. Documentation is more vital than ever before, and patient care cannot be legally justified without documentation of the effectiveness of treatment for the patient.

REFERENCES

1. Magee David J. *Orthopedic Physical Assessment.*3rd ed. Philadelphia: W.B. Saunders; 1997.
2. MacNab I, McCulloch J. *Bachache.*2nd ed. Baltimore: Williams& Wilkins; 1990.
3. Seidel H, Ball J, Dains J, Benedict GW. *Mosby's Guide to Physical Exam.* 3rd ed. St. Louis: Mosby; 1995.
4. Bovee M. *The Essentials of the Orthopedic & Neurologic Exam.* Self-Published; 1977.
5. Swartz M. *TextBook of Physical Diagnosis History and Exam.* Philadelphia: W.B. Saunders; 1989.
6. Cohn R. Ernest. *Impairment Rating Examination and Disability Evaluation.* Self-Published Course Notes; 1995.
7. Farfan H.F. The scientific basis of manipulative procedures. *Clinics in Rheumatic Diseases.* 1980; Vol. 6. 1:159-173
8. Markey L.Paul. *Managing Disorders of the Lumbar Spine.* 2nd ed. Self-Published; 1986.
9. Foreman, Stephen and Croft, Arthur C.: *Whiplash Injuries: Taking the Pain Out of Personal Injury* (Tape Series). Listen & Learn Publ., 1990.
10. Baechle T. *Essentials of Strength and Conditioning.* Champaign: Human Kinetics; 1994.
11. Gerard J.A, Kleinfield S.L. *Orthopaedic Testing.* New York: Churchill-Livingstone; 1993.
12 Mennell, John McM.: *The Musculoskeletal System: Differential Diagnosis from Symptoms and Physical Signs.* An Aspen Publication, 1992.
13. Souza T.A. Which orthopedic tests are really necessary? In: Lawrence DJ, Cassidy JD, McGreagor M, et al., eds. *Advances in Chiropractic.* St. Louis, MO: Mosby-Year Book; 1994;1:101-158.
14. Yochum, Terry R. and Rowe, Lindsay J.: *Essentials of Skeletal Radiology.* 2nd ed., Vol. 1; Williams & Wilkins. 1996.
15. DeMyer W. *Technique of the Neurologic Exam: A Programmed Text.* 4th ed. New York: McGraw-Hill; 1994.
16. Goldberg S. *The Four-Minute Neurologic Exam.* Miami: Medmaster; 1988.
17. Hoppenfeld S. *Orthopedic Neurology.* Philadelphia: J.B. Lippincott; 1977.
18. Ferezy J. *The Chiropractic Neurologic Exam.* Gaithersburg: Aspen; 1992.
19. Maitland GD. The slump test: examination and treatment. *The Australian Journal of Physiotherapy.* 1985; Vol. 31 No. 6.
20. Miller, K. Jeffrey. The slump test: Clinical applications and interpretations. *Chiropractic Technique.* 1999; Vol. 11 No. 4.
21. American Medical Association. *Guides to the Evaluation of Permanent Impairment.* 3rd ed. Chicago: AMA; 1988.
22. American Medical Association. *Guides to the Evaluation of Permanent Impairment.* 4th ed. Chicago: AMA; 1988.
23. Blauvelt, Carolyn Taliaferro and Nelson, Fred RT.: *A Manual of Orthopaedic Terminology.* Fourth Edition. The C.V.Mosby Company, 1990.
24. Junghanns H. *Clinical Implications of Normal Biomechanical Stresses on Spinal Function.* Gaithersberg: Aspen; 1990.
25. Netter F. *Low Back Pain.* Summit: CIBA Clinical Symposia Vol. 32 No. 6; 1980.
26. Ramamurti C.P. *Orthopedics in Primary Care.* Baltimore: Williams & Wilkins; 1979.
27. Miller, K. Jeffrey. Patrick's test and Sacroiliac pathology. *Orthopedic Brief.* June; 1997.
28. Herron L.D., Pheasant HC. Prone knee-flexion provocative testing for lumbar disc protrusion. *Spine.* 1980;1:65-67.
29. *Adjusting Technique Manual.* Technique Department, Palmer College of Chiropractic. Palmer College of Chiropractic, 1995.
30. Nachemson A.L. The lumbar spine: an orthopedic challenge. *Spine.* 1976;1:59-71.
31. Bates B. *A Guide to Physical Exam.* 3rd ed. Philadelphia: J.B. Lippincott; 1983.

Appendix A

Practical Examination Strategies:

1. Patient history should precede examination.

2. The examination performed should be based on or related to the history obtained prior to the exam.

3. Positive results of orthopedic and neurological exam procedures should be recorded according to their intended meanings or interpretations.

4. Exam findings should be easy to record.

5. Exam results should be easy for third parties to read.

6. Exam procedures and the records of the procedures should protect the doctor/practice should accusations of malpractice arise.

7. A routine examination should be easy to perform and time-efficient.

8. Exam procedures should not be limited to tests related solely to a specific chiropractic technique.

9. Exam procedures in chiropractic practice should be applicable to patients with a variety of complaints related to the head, spine, pelvis and extremities.

10. The procedures utilized during examination should be well-accepted and widely used.

11. Exam techniques should seek to identify or rule out ominous conditions and contraindications to chiropractic adjustment.

12. Exams should minimize discomfort for the patient.

13. The examination process should take advantage of overlapping body mechanics among procedures. Combining maneuvers increases efficiency.

14. An unremarkable or an inappropriate response to tests used in combination usually indicates that all tests in that group are negative.

15. A positive response to any test that has been performed in combination with other tests may indicate a need to perform each test in the group individually.

16. Tests that confirm or reinforce the results of other tests should be included in the examination process.

17. Testing procedures, which can be performed utilizing more than one patient position, should be performed first in the position most likely to produce positive results.

18. The examination process should include methods for identifying malingering and non-organic conditions.

19. Physical examination procedures should establish the reasoning behind ordering or not ordering additional tests, such as imaging or lab studies.

20. Exam procedures should be applicable for both new and established patient evaluations.

Appendix B

History and Exam Forms

WELCOME! Please allow our staff to photocopy your driver's license and all available insurance cards.

PLEASE PRINT.

Full Name _____ Gender: **M F** Home Phone_____

Address _____City _____ State _____Zip_____

Age _____Birth Date _____ Marital Status (Circle One): **S M W D Sep** No. Children _____

SS#_____ Driver's License # _____

Your Employer _____Your Occupation_____Years on Job _____

Employer Address_____City _____ State _____Zip_____

Work Phone_____

Do you have health insurance where you work? ❑ Yes ❑ No Plan/Group # _____

Insurance Company_____

Name of Spouse, Parent or Guardian _____ Age _____ Birth Date _____ SS#_____

Spouse's Employer _____Spouse's Occupation_____Years on Job _____

Employer Address_____City _____ State _____Zip_____

Work Phone_____

Does your spouse have health insurance at work? ❑ Yes ❑ No Plan/Group # _____

Insurance Company_____

How did you find out about our office? _____

Describe the major complaints that brought you to our office:_____

_____

Is your condition due to an accident? ❑ Yes ❑ No Date of accident: _____

I (we) agree to pay for services rendered to the above-mentioned patient as the charge is incurred. I (we) understand that health and accident insurance policies are arrangements between an insurance carrier and myself and that I am personally responsible for payment of any and all services, covered or non-covered. If the doctor is a contracted provider for my managed care plan, I understand I am responsible for all copayments and non-covered services. I also understand and agree to pay all copays and fees for non-covered services prior to seeing the doctor. I understand that if I terminate my care and treatment, any fees for professional services rendered me will be immediately due and payable. I understand that unpaid fees for services beyond thirty (30) days are subject to a 1.5% monthly finance charge (18% annually).

I (we) authorize the doctor and his staff to release any information deemed appropriate concerning my physical condition to any insurance company, claims adjuster, case nurse, claims reviewer, employer, health care provider or attorney in order to process any claim for reimbursement or charges incurred by me as a result of professional services rendered and hereby release him/her of any consequences thereof. I agree that a photostatic copy of this agreement shall serve as the original.

I (we) hereby authorize and direct payment of any medical/chiropractic expense benefits allowable to the doctor as payment toward the total charges for professional services rendered. This payment will not exceed my indebtedness to the assignee. I agree that a photostatic copy of this agreement shall serve as the original.

Patient's Signature_____ Date _____

Spouse's or Guardian's Signature _____ Date _____

We file your primary insurance at no charge to you. Filings for policies in addition to your primary coverage are completed *for a fee and as time permits.*

Payment Options (Please Indicate): ❑ Cash ❑ Check ❑ MasterCard ❑ Visa ❑ Discover

NAME_____ DATE _____

AGE_____ OCCUPATION_____

RACE: ❑ Cauc. ❑ Black ❑ Hisp. ❑ Asian ❑ Am. Indian ❑ Other_____Sex ❑ M ❑ F

PATIENT/INFORMANT STATES: _____

_____

_____

DETAILS OF CHIEF COMPLAINT: DOCTOR'S NOTES:

1. **Location of Symptoms/Dysfunction:**   1. Points To:_____

In order of onset: 1 _____2 _____3 _____4 _____   _____

Intensity of pain: _____ _____ _____ _____   _____

(Patient's perception)   _____

AMA Scale: Minimal 1-3, Slight 4-6, Moderate 7-9, Marked 10   _____

Borg Scale: Normal 0, Low 1-3, Moderate 4-6, Intense 7-9, Emergency 10   _____

2. **Radiation/Spread/Referral of Pain:** ❑ Y   ❑ N   2._____

3. **Onset:**_____   3._____
When did it start?   _____
Explanation: _____   _____
How did it start?   _____
❑ WC   ❑ PI   ❑ MM   ❑ MC   ❑ C   ❑ PA   _____

_____

Date of First Report:_____ Date of First Visit: _____   _____

4. **Type of Sensation:** _____   4._____

Quality of pain?/What does it feel like?   _____

5. **Frequency (Timing):**   5._____

❑ Intermit. 0-25 ❑ Occas. 26- 50 ❑ Frequent 51-75 ❑ Constant 76-100   _____

6. **Exacerbation/Aggravation/Increase:** ❑ Y   ❑ N   6._____

Postures, activity, time of day, etc.

7. **Symptoms/Dysfunction Since Onset Have:**   7._____

❑ Decreased ❑ Increased ❑ Remained About The Same ❑ Erratic   _____

8. **Change In Bodily Functions:** ❑ Y   ❑ N   8._____

❑ Balance	❑ Bowel Habits	❑ Breathing	❑ Coordination
❑ Coughing	❑ Gait	❑ Grip	❑ Hearing
❑ Menstrual	❑ Sexual	❑ Sleep	❑ Sneezing
❑ Urination	❑ Vision	❑ Weakness	❑ Weight

_____

9. **Handedness:** ❑ L   ❑ R   ❑ Am.   9._____

Case # _____

Page 3 of _____

10. **Change In Activities of Daily Living:** ❑ Y ❑ N

What do you not do because of this problem?

❑ Forgotten with activity ❑ Interferes with activity ❑ Activity continues

❑ May prevent activity ❑ Prevents activity   despite problem

10. _____
_____
_____
_____
_____

11. **Work Status: No. of Jobs 1 2 3**

❑ Full-time   ❑ Part-time   ❑ Homemaker   ❑ Student

❑ Retired   ❑ Disabled   ❑ Unemployed   ❑ Shift 1 2 3

11._____
_____
_____

12. **Work/Home Disability:** ❑ Y ❑ N

Complete: _____ Days off work

_____ Days unable to perform household tasks

Partial: _____ Days of job modification

_____ Days of decreased household tasks

12._____
_____
_____
_____
_____

13. **Store-bought or Home Remedies:** ❑ Y ❑ N

Care not recommended by a doctor.

Type/Effect:_____

13._____
- -
- -

14. **Other Professional Care:** ❑ Y ❑ N

Type, Tests, Dx, Tx, Effect:_____

_____
_____
_____

14._____
_____
_____
_____

15. **Remission/Relief/Decrease:** ❑ Y ❑ N

Postures, activities, time of day, etc.

15._____
_____
_____

16. **Same or Similar Condition:** ❑ Y ❑ N

Explanation: _____

_____
_____

16._____
_____
_____
_____

17. **Concurrent Symptoms/Conditions:** ❑ Y ❑ N

Are you currently under a doctor's care for any other condition(s)?

17._____
_____

18. **Do You Have A Pacemaker or Any Other**
Surgically Implanted Device? ❑ Y ❑ N

18._____
_____

19. **Are You Now or Could You Be Pregnant?** ❑ Y ❑ N

19._____
_____

CASE HISTORY

Please answer the questions below concerning your health history. Be sure to list all conditions or symptoms, both past or present.

An understanding of your health history will help us to determine appropriate care.

FULL NAME _____ DATE _____ CASE # _____

AGE _____ RACE _____ GENDER _____ HEIGHT _____ WEIGHT _____

Review of Systems

1. Do you have skin, hair or nail problems? ❑ Yes ❑ No _____
2. Do you have mouth and/or throat problems? ❑ Yes ❑ No _____
3. Do you have nose and/or sinus problems? ❑ Yes ❑ No _____
4. Do you have ear problems? ❑ Yes ❑ No _____
5. Do you have eye problems? ❑ Yes ❑ No _____
6. Do you have chest or lung (breathing) problems? ❑ Yes ❑ No _____
7. Do you smoke? ❑ Yes ❑ No Cigarettes per day _____ How Long? _____
8. Do you have heart and/or blood vessel problems? ❑ Yes ❑ No _____
9. Do you have blood or lymph node problems? ❑ Yes ❑ No _____
10. Do you have digestive problems? ❑ Yes ❑ No _____
11. Do you have genital problems (e.g., prostate, testicular, vaginal)? ❑ Yes ❑ No _____
12. Do you have urinary (including kidney or bladder) problems? ❑ Yes ❑ No _____
13. **Females**, have you had menstrual problems? ❑ Yes ❑ No _____
    Have you ever taken birth control pills? ❑ Yes ❑ No For how long? _____
    Is there any chance that you are currently pregnant? ❑ Yes ❑ No
    Do you have any breast problems? ❑ Yes ❑ No _____
14. Do you have any nervous system diseases and/or mental health problems? ❑ Yes ❑ No
    _____
15. Do you have any gland and/or hormone problems? ❑ Yes ❑ No _____
16. Do you have allergy or immuity problems? ❑ Yes ❑ No _____
17. Do you have any muscle, tendon or ligament problems? ❑ Yes ❑ No _____
18. Do you have any bone or joint diseases (examples: bone = osteoporosis, joint = arthritis)? ❑ Yes ❑ No _____
    _____

Past History

19. List any diseases that you have had in the past, including childhood diseases: _____
    _____
20. Tell us if you have ever been diagnosed as having a particular condition, such as diabetes, cancer, AIDS, etc.: _____
    _____
21. Have you suffered any physical injuries, such as falls or blows, automobile accidents, whiplash, concussion or head injury, lacerations, sprains, strains, dislocations, broken or cracked bones? ❑ Yes ❑ No
    _____
    _____
22. List any surgeries you have had (don't forget appendix, tonsils, ear tubes, wisdom teeth):
    _____ Date _____
    _____ Date _____
    _____ Date _____
    _____ Date _____

(OVER PLEASE)

FULL NAME _____ DATE _____ CASE # _____

23. Have you ever been hospitalized for any reason other than surgery? ❑ Yes ❑ No _____

24. **Medications:** Please list all medications (prescription & non-prescription) you are currently taking or take on an occasional basis:_____
_____

25. Your diet is: ❑ Balanced ❑ Fair ❑ Poor ❑ Excessive ❑ Restricted

Family History

26. Are there any diseases or conditions that are common among your family members (i.e., inherited diseases or conditions)? ❑ Yes ❑ No _____

Social History

27. In what position do you usually sleep, and how well? _____
_____

28. Do you exercise on a regular basis? ❑ Yes ❑ No How? _____

29. How do you spend your spare time (hobbies, etc)?_____

30. Do you use: ❑ Caffein? ❑ Tobacco? ❑ Nicotine? ❑ Recreational Drugs? ❑ Alcohol?

31. Please describe your work.

   Type: ❑ Professional ❑ Physical Labor ❑ Driver ❑ Clerical ❑ Factory ❑ Homemaker

   Physical Demands: ❑ Heavy ❑ Moderate ❑ Mild ❑ Sedentary

   Stress Level: ❑ High ❑ Medium ❑ Low

Additional Questions

32. Do you have problems with recurring headaches? ❑ Yes ❑ No _____

33. Are you losing weight without trying? ❑ Yes ❑ No

34. Does your pain wake you up at night? ❑ Yes ❑ No

35. Have you had a change in bowel or bladder habits? ❑ Yes ❑ No _____

36. Have you had a sore that doesn't heal? ❑ Yes ❑ No _____

37. Have you recently had any unusual bleeding or discharge? ❑ Yes ❑ No _____

38. Do you have a thickening/lump in the breast or elsewhere? ❑ Yes ❑ No _____

39. Do you have indigestion or difficulty swallowing? ❑ Yes ❑ No _____

40. Have you had an obvious change in a wart or mole? ❑ Yes ❑ No _____

41. Do you have a nagging cough or hoarseness? ❑ Yes ❑ No _____

42. In the space below, please explain or give additional details regarding the information you have given above. Also, if there is any information about your health history that was not requested, please fill it in below.
_____
_____

43. Please describe your current complaint. In other words, what brought you here? _____
_____
_____

44. Who is your:

   Medical Doctor? _____

   OB/GYN? _____

   Dentist? _____

NAME _____ AGE _____ DATE _____ CASE # _____

Have you ever (at any time) experienced any of the following?

Difficulty urinating	Y	N	Claustrophobia (fear of small spaces)	Y	N
Loss of bladder control	Y	N	Spinal surgery	Y	N
Loss of bowel control	Y	N	Common cold/flu	Y	N
Temporary loss of vision, one eye	Y	N	Carotid artery surgery	Y	N
Blood in urine	Y	N	Breast removal	Y	N

Have you ever been diagnosed with or told you have one of the following?

Detached retina	Y	N	Rheumatoid arthritis	Y	N
Stroke	Y	N	Fractured/broken vertebra	Y	N
Slipped disc	Y	N	Bleeding disorders	Y	N
Herniated disc	Y	N	High blood pressure	Y	N
Osteoporosis	Y	N	Blood in stool	Y	N
TIAís (pin or mini strokes)	Y	N	Cancer	Y	N
Drop attacks (collapsing, but not fainting)	Y	N	AIDS	Y	N
Hardening of the arteries	Y	N	Kidney disease	Y	N
Partial or complete paralysis	Y	N	Prostate disease	Y	N

Do you currently have, or could you be, any of the following?

Pregnant	Y	N
Taking birth control pills	Y	N
Receiving hormone therapy	Y	N
Male Female		
Receiving chemotherapy	Y	N
Receiving radiation therapy	Y	N
Taking blood thinners	Y	N
A heavy smoker (1 or more packs/ day)	Y	N
Surgical/medical implanted devices:		
Aortic clips	Y	N
Brain clips	Y	N
Artificial heart valves	Y	N
Rods, pins, screws	Y	N
IUD	Y	N
Surgical clips/wires	Y	N
Shunt	Y	N
Neurostimulator	Y	N
Dentures	Y	N
Pacemaker	Y	N
Hearing aid	Y	N
Insulin pump	Y	N
Joint replacement	Y	N
Cochlear implants (ear)	Y	N
Other implanted devices:		
Metal fragments (head, eye, skin)	Y	N
Bullets/shrapnel	Y	N
Body piercing	Y	N
Tattoos	Y	N

In the past 14 days, have you experienced any of the following?

Nausea	Y	N
Vomiting	Y	N
Vertigo (spinning)	Y	N
Difficulty walking	Y	N
Incoordination	Y	N
Numbness or other sensory complaints	Y	N
Loss of consciousness	Y	N
Double vision	Y	N
Blurred vision	Y	N
Tinnitus (ringing in ears)	Y	N
Speech problems	Y	N
Clumsiness	Y	N
Memory loss	Y	N
Travel by car/truck	Y	N
Personality changes	Y	N
Fever	Y	N
Recurrent headaches	Y	N
Diarrhea	Y	N
Used a tanning bed/booth	Y	N
Skin rash/infection	Y	N
A major fall	Y	N
A minor fall	Y	N
An auto accident	Y	N
A work injury	Y	N
Loss of strength	Y	N
Pain during bowel movements	Y	N
Head trauma	Y	N
Abnormal period	Y	N

NAME _____ AGE_____ DATE _____ CASE # _____

DO YOU CURRENTLY HAVE ANY OF THE FOLLOWING?

Integument System

Skin rash	Y	N
Skin lesion	Y	N
Changes in skin color	Y	N
Itching (pruritus)	Y	N
Hair changes	Y	N
Nail changes	Y	N

Endocrine System

Hormone problems	Y	N
Hot flashes	Y	N
Thyroid problems	Y	N
Hormone therapy	Y	N
Growth abnormalities	Y	N
Metabolism changes	Y	N

Digestive System

Abdominal pain	Y	N
Nausea	Y	N
Vomiting	Y	N
Constipation	Y	N
Diarrhea	Y	N

Rectal bleeding	Y	N
Jaundice	Y	N
Abdominal distention	Y	N
Cramping	Y	N
Lump/mass	Y	N

Cardiovascular System

Chest pain	Y	N
Irregular heartbeat	Y	N
Shortness of breath	Y	N
Fainting	Y	N
Fatigue	Y	N
Swelling of legs	Y	N

Changes in skin color	Y	N
Stroke (full or pin)	Y	N
Dizziness	Y	N
Cool hands or feet	Y	N
Varicose veins	Y	N
Mitral valve problems	Y	N

Pulmonary System

Coughing	Y	N
Phlegm/expectorant	Y	N
Coughing up blood	Y	N
Shortness of breath	Y	N
Wheezing	Y	N
Blue skin (cyanosis)	Y	N
Chest pain	Y	N

Musculoskeletal System

Stiffness	Y	N
Popping noises	Y	N
Joint pain	Y	N
Weakness	Y	N
Limitation of movement	Y	N
Extremity deformities	Y	N
Difficulty walking	Y	N

Nervous System

Partial paralysis	Y	N
Complete paralysis	Y	N
Headache	Y	N
Are you right-handed?	Y	N
Loss of consciousness	Y	N
Dizziness	Y	N
Memory loss	Y	N
Numbness	Y	N
Weakness	Y	N
Depression	Y	N

Lack of coordination	Y	N
Psychiatric disorders	Y	N
Speech abnormalities	Y	N
Visual disturbances	Y	N
Are you left-handed?	Y	N
Gait disorders	Y	N
Tremors	Y	N
Tics (spasms)	Y	N
Sensory changes	Y	N
Mood changes	Y	N

(CONTINUED)

NAME _____ AGE_____ DATE _____ CASE # _____

Genital/Urinary System

Pain during urination	Y	N
Changes in urine flow	Y	N
Lump or mass in groin	Y	N
Kidney stones	Y	N
Chronic bladder infections	Y	N
Genital itching	Y	N
Changes in urination frequency	Y	N
Change in urine color	Y	N

Special Senses

Visual problems	Y	N
Hearing loss	Y	N
Loss of balance	Y	N
Loss of taste	Y	N
Loss of smell	Y	N
Loss of touch sensation	Y	N
Temporary vision loss in one eye	Y	N

Reproductive System

Male Only

Testicular pain	Y	N
Prostate problems	Y	N
Infertility	Y	N
Impotence	Y	N
Discharge	Y	N
Lump or mass	Y	N

Female Only

Abnormal vaginal bleeding	Y	N
Painful menstruation	Y	N
Breast lump/mass	Y	N
Vaginal discharge/itching	Y	N
Nipple discharge	Y	N
Infertility	Y	N
Abnormal periods	Y	N
Male pattern baldness	Y	N

Head and Neck Region

Headaches	Y	N	Ringing in ears	Y	N
Neck stiffness	Y	N	Ear pain	Y	N
Neck lump/mass	Y	N	Ear discharge	Y	N
Eye pain	Y	N	Ear itching	Y	N
Eye redness	Y	N	Nasal discharge	Y	N
Eye discharge	Y	N	Sinus trouble	Y	N
Double vision	Y	N	Bad breath	Y	N
Dry eyes	Y	N	Nasal obstruction	Y	N
Excessive tearing	Y	N	Snoring	Y	N
Spinning sensation	Y	N			

Blood, Lymphatics, Immunology, Allergy

Anemia	Y	N	Frequent illness	Y	N
Iron deficiency	Y	N	Immunity problems	Y	N
Clotting problems	Y	N	Allergies	Y	N
Bruise easily	Y	N	Take allergy shots	Y	N
Swollen lymph nodes	Y	N			

Doctor's Notes

_____

_____

_____

_____

EXAMINATION FINDINGS
PAGE # 1

PATIENT: _____ DATE: _____ CASE # _____

Group #1

STANDING	SEATED			SEATED		
HEIGHT / WEIGHT		BLOOD PRESSURE mmHg		TEMPERATURE		HANDEDNESS

ft	in		lb	R		L	F		Left	Ambi	Right

OBSERVATIONS

Group #2

MOOD	Pleasant		Calm		Depressed		Anxious		Agitated	
ORIENTATION	Person			Place			Time			
	ABN	WNL		ABN	WNL		ABN	WNL		
BODY TYPE	Ectomorph			Endomorph			Mesomorph			
GROOMING	Poor			Fair			Good			

Group #3

ANTALGIA	Head	C-spine	T-spine	L-spine	Pelvis	UE	LE		Pos	Neg
MINORS		Pos		Neg	FORWARD-HEAD		Pos			Neg
LUM-HYPER		Pos		Neg	LUM-HYPO		Pos			Neg
SPINAL ERECTORS							Weak	Tight		WNL
ABDOMINAL MUSCLES							Weak	Tight		WNL
HAMSTRINGS		Left		Right	Bilateral		Weak	Tight		WNL
QUADRICEPS		Left		Right	Bilateral		Weak	Tight		WNL
HIP FLEXORS		Left		Right	Bilateral		Weak	Tight		WNL
ILIOTIBIAL BAND		Left		Right	Bilateral		Weak	Tight		WNL

SEATED

Group #4

CAROTID BRUIT	Left	Right	Bilateral	Pos	Neg
HAUTANT	Left	Right	Bilateral	Pos	Neg
DRIFT	Left	Right	Bilateral	Pos	Neg
FINGER-TO-NOSE	Left	Right	Bilateral	Pos	Neg
CERV COMPRESSION	Left	Right	Bilateral	Pos	Neg
CERV DISTRACTION	Left	Right	Bilateral	Pos	Neg

Group #5

HAND GRASP	Left	Right	Bilateral	Abnormal	WNL
HOFFMAN	Left	Right	Bilateral	Present	Absent

Group #6

BICEPS	Left	Right	Bilateral	Absent	Hypo	Hyper	Symmetrical	WNL
BRACHIO-RADIALIS	Left	Right	Bilateral	Absent	Hypo	Hyper	Symmetrical	WNL
TRICEPS	Left	Right	Bilateral	Absent	Hypo	Hyper	Symmetrical	WNL

(CONTINUED)

81

PATIENT: _____ DATE: _____ CASE # _____

		Left	Central	Right	Spine	SI	UE	LE	Mus	Neuro	Pos	Neg
Group #7	SLUMP										Pos	Neg
	SOTO-HALL										Pos	Neg
	LINDNER										Pos	Neg
	LHERMETTE										Pos	Neg
	BRUDZINSKI										Pos	Neg
	BECHTEREW										Pos	Neg
	SLR										Pos	Neg
	CSLR										Pos	Neg
	TRIPOD										Pos	Neg
	KERNIG										Pos	Neg
	BRAGGARD										Pos	Neg
	FAJERSZTAJN										Pos	Neg
	VALSALVA										Pos	Neg
	DEJERINE										Pos	Neg

SEATED

	Cervical ROM	Measured	Observed	Aberrant Motion		Crepitus		Pain		WNL
Group #8	FLEXION			Pos	Neg	Pos	Neg	Pos	Neg	50
	EXTENSION			Pos	Neg	Pos	Neg	Pos	Neg	60
	RIGHT LATERAL FLEXION			Pos	Neg	Pos	Neg	Pos	Neg	45
	LEFT LATERAL FLEXION			Pos	Neg	Pos	Neg	Pos	Neg	45
	RIGHT ROTATION			Pos	Neg	Pos	Neg	Pos	Neg	80
	LEFT ROTATION			Pos	Neg	Pos	Neg	Pos	Neg	80

SUPPLEMENTARY PROCEDURES: _____ **Use of this section not indicated**

Group #9	BRACHIO PLEXUS	Left	Right	Bilateral	Pos	Neg
	BAKODY	Left	Right	Bilateral	Pos	Neg

SUPPLEMENTARY PROCEDURES: _____ **Use of this section not indicated**

Group #10	ADSON	Left	Right	Bilateral	Pos	Neg
	HALSTEAD	Left	Right	Bilateral	Pos	Neg
	EDENS	Left	Right	Bilateral	Pos	Neg
	WRIGHT	Left	Right	Bilateral	Pos	Neg
	GEORGE'S FUNCTIONAL	Left	Right	Bilateral	Pos	Neg

(CONTINUED)

PATIENT: _____ DATE: _____ CASE # _____

STANDING

Group #11

KNEE BENDS(5)		Left	Right	Bilateral	Abnormal	WNL
	Hip Flex L2-L3	Hip Ext L4-L5	Knee Ext L3-L4	Knee Flex L5-S1	Ank Dorsi L4-L5	Ank Plan S1-S2
CREPITUS						
TOE RAISES(25)	S1-S2	Left	Right	Bilateral	Abnormal	WNL
HEEL STANDING	L4	Left	Right	Bilateral	Abnormal	WNL
TANDEM STANCE	Coordination				Abnormal	WNL

Group #12

Lumbosacral ROM	Measured	Observed	Aberrant Motion		Crepitus		Pain		WNL
FLEXION			Pos	Neg	Pos	Neg	Pos	Neg	60
EXTENSION			Pos	Neg	Pos	Neg	Pos	Neg	25
RIGHT LATERAL FLEXION			Pos	Neg	Pos	Neg	Pos	Neg	25
LEFT LATERAL FLEXION			Pos	Neg	Pos	Neg	Pos	Neg	25

PRONE

Group #13

HIBBS	Left	Right	Bilateral	Pos	Neg
SPHINX	Left	Right	Central	Pos	Neg
NACHLAS	Left SI	Right SI	L/S	Pos	Neg
FEMORAL STRETCH	Left	Right	Bilateral	Pos	Neg
PRONE KNEE FLEXION	Left	Right	Bilateral	Pos	Neg

Group #14

ACHILLES	Left	Right	Bilateral	Absent	Hypo	Hyper	Symetrical	WNL
PATELLAR	Left	Right	Bilateral	Absent	Hypo	Hyper	Symetrical	WNL
BABINSKI	Left	Right	Bilateral	Present		Absent		

PRONE PALPATION

Group #15

CERVICAL	Joint Dysfunction									Joint Dysfunction	
	Level	0	1	2	3	4	5	6	7	WNL	
	Muscle Tone									Muscle Tone	

KEY
Joint: Left Ⓛ,
Right Ⓡ or
Bilateral Ⓑ

THORACIC	Joint Dysfunction													Joint Dysfunction
	Level		1	2	3	4	5	6	7	8	9	10	11	12	WNL
	Muscle Tone													Muscle Tone

LUMBAR	Joint Dysfunction						Joint Dysfunction
	Level		1	2	3	4	5	WNL
	Muscle Tone						Muscle Tone

KEY
Muscle: Hypertonicity (↑)
or Hypotonicity (↓)

PELVIC	Fluid Motion	Left SI	Right SI	POS	NEG

(CONTINUED)

85

PATIENT: _____ DATE: _____ CASE # _____

SUPINE
SUPPLEMENTARY PROCEDURES: _____ **Use of this section not indicated**

		Left	Central	Right	Spine	SI	UE	LE	Mus	Neuro	Pos	Neg
Group #16	SOTO-HALL										Pos	Neg
	LINDNER										Pos	Neg
	LHERMETTE										Pos	Neg
	BRUDZINSKI										Pos	Neg
	SLR										Pos	Neg
	CSLR										Pos	Neg
	KERNIG										Pos	Neg
	BRAGGARD										Pos	Neg
	FAJERSZTAJN										Pos	Neg
	VALSALVA										Pos	Neg
	DEJERINE										Pos	Neg

SUPPLEMENTARY PROCEDURES: _____ **Use of this section not indicated.**

Group #17	RADIAL PULSE	Left	Absent	Weak	Strong	Right	Absent	Weak	Strong
	POST TIBIAL	Left	Absent	Weak	Strong	Right	Absent	Weak	Strong

NOTES: _____

_____

_____

_____

_____

_____

_____

_____

SUMMARY: _____

_____

_____

_____

_____

_____

WORKING Dx:_____ DDx: _____ Initial/Sign: _____

Appendix C

Functions, Pathologies and
Corresponding Tests and Signs

1. **ANTALGIC POSTURING:** Observation.

2. **BODY TYPE:** Height, observation, weight.

3. **CAROTID BRUITS:** Auscultation.

4. **CENTRAL NERVOUS SYSTEM DYSFUNCTION:** Babinski, Brudzinski, drift, finger-to-nose, Hoffman's, hyper deep tendon reflexes, Kernig, Lhermette's, orientation, tandem stance.

5. **CREPITUS:** All spinal and extremity ranges of motion.

6. **COORDINATION:** Finger-to-nose, tandem stance.

7. **DEEP TENDON REFLEXES:** Achilles, biceps, brachiaoradialis, patellar, triceps.

8. **DISC PATHOLOGIES:** Bakody's, Bechterew's, brachial plexus, Braggard's, cervical compression, cervical distraction, CSLR, Dejerine, Fajersztajn, femoral stretch, Lindner's, SLR, slump, Valsalva.

9. **FACET SYNDROME:** Nachlas, Sphinx.

10. **FEVER:** Temperature.

11. **HEIGHT:** Height measurement.

12. **HIP (COXA) JOINT PATHOLOGIES:** Hibbs.

13. **HYPERTENSION:** Blood pressure.

14. **INFECTIONS:** Brudzinski, Kernig (see meningitis), temperature.

15. **JOINT FIXATION:** Palpation, fluid motion test.

16. **LOWER EXTREMITY MOTOR FUNCTION:** Drift, heel standing, knee bends, toe raises.

17. **LOWER EXTREMITY RANGE OF MOTION:** Knee bends.

18. **MALINGERING:** Lying versus seated SLR (Bechterew's), tripod.

19. **MENINGITIS:** Brudzinski, Kernig, temperature.

20. **MUSCLE IMBALANCE:** Observation for antalgia, Minors sign, forward head posture, lumbar hyperlordosis, lumbar hypolordosis, hamstring tension, quadriceps tension, hip flexor tension, iliotibial band tension, spinal erectors, abdominal muscles.

21. **MUSCLE TONE:** Crepitus, palpation, range of motion, motor function, various orthopedic maneuvers.

22. **NEUROMENINGEAL TRACT TENSION:** Slump.

23. **NERVE ROOT TENSION:** Bakody, Bechterew's, brachial plexus, Braggard's, cervical compression, cervical distraction, CSLR, Fajersztajn's, femoral stretch, Lindner's, SLR, slump.

24. **ORIENTATION:** Person, place, time.

25. **PATHOLOGICAL REFLEXES:** Babinski, Hoffman.

26. **PERIPHERAL NERVOUS DYSFUNCTION:** Deep tendon reflexes, disc pathology, motor function, nerve root tension, thoracic outlet syndrome and spinal/pelvic subluxation.

27. **PERIPHERAL VASCULAR COMPROMISE:** Adson, Eden's, Halstead, posterior tibial pulse, radial pulse, Wright's.

28. **POSTURE/STATION:** Observation for antalgia, Minors sign, forward head posture, lumbar hyperlordosis, lumbar hypolordosis, hamstring tension, quadriceps tension, hip flexor tension, iliotibial band tension, spinal erectors, abdominal muscles.

29. **SACROILIAC JOINT DYSFUNCTION:** Fluid motion test, Nachlas, palpation, slump.

30. **SPACE OCCUPYING LESION:** Dejerine, Valsalva.

31. **SPINAL CORD PATHOLOGY:** Deep tendon reflexes (see #7), Lhermette, pathological reflexes (see #25).

32. **SPINAL RANGE OF MOTION:** Direct exam or see Table 8.

33. **SPINAL STENOSIS:** Prone knee flexion, sphinx.

34. **SPRAINS (LIGAMENT):** Nachlas, palpation, Soto-Hall.

35. **STRAINS (MUSCLE):** Palpation, Soto-Hall.

36. **SUBLUXATION:** Fluid motion test, palpation, range of motion.

37. **THORACIC OUTLET SYNDROMES:** Adson, Eden's, Halstead, Wright's.

38. **UPPER EXTREMITY MOTOR FUNCTION:** Drift, hand grasp.

39. **UPPER MOTOR NEURON LESIONS:** DTR's (see #7), pathological reflexes (see #25).

40. **VERTEBRAL ARTERY COMPROMISE:** George's Functional Maneuver, Hautant's.

41. **WEIGHT:** Weight measurement.